PRENTICE-HALL

FOUNDATIONS OF IMMUNOLOGY SERIES

EDITORS

Abraham G. Osler

*The Public Health Research Institute of the City of New York
and New York University School of Medicine*

Leon Weiss

The Johns Hopkins University School of Medicine

THE IMMUNOBIOLOGY OF TRANSPLANTATION
Rupert E. Billingham and Willys Silvers

THE CELLS AND TISSUES OF THE IMMUNE SYSTEM
Leon Weiss

COMPLEMENT: MECHANISMS AND FUNCTIONS
Abraham G. Osler

THE IMMUNE SYSTEM OF SECRETION
Thomas B. Tomasi, Jr.

COMPARATIVE IMMUNOLOGY
Edwin L. Cooper

THE IMMUNOBIOLOGY OF MAMMALIAN REPRODUCTION
Alan E. Beer and Rupert E. Billingham

RADIOIMMUNOASSAY OF BIOLOGICALLY ACTIVE COMPOUNDS
Charles W. Parker

COMPLEMENT
Mechanisms and Functions

ABRAHAM G. OSLER, Ph.D.

*The Public Health Research Institute
of the City of New York*

PRENTICE-HALL, INC., *Englewood Cliffs, N.J.*

Library of Congress Cataloging in Publication Data

OSLER, ABRAHAM G. (date)
Complement.

(Prentice-Hall foundations of immunology series)
Includes bibliographies and index.
1. Complements (Immunity)   I. Title.
QR185.8.C6084   616.07'9   75-15982
ISBN   0-13-155226-0

10   9   8   7   6   5   4   3   2   1

PRINTED IN THE UNITED STATES OF AMERICA

PRENTICE-HALL INTERNATIONAL, INC., *London*
PRENTICE-HALL OF AUSTRALIA, PTY. LTD., *Sydney*
PRENTICE-HALL OF CANADA, LTD., *Toronto*
PRENTICE-HALL OF INDIA PRIVATE LIMITED, *New Delhi*
PRENTICE-HALL OF JAPAN, INC., *Tokyo*
PRENTICE-HALL OF SOUTHEAST ASIA (PTE.) LTD., *Singapore*

To

SONIA

Foundations of Immunology Series

This series of monographs is intended to provide readers of diverse backgrounds with an authoritative and clear statement concerning significant aspects of immunology. Each volume represents an individual contribution by a distinguished scientist. As a series, they provide a comprehensive view of the field.

The editors have encouraged the individuality of each author in content and method of presentation. They have sought as the major objective of the series, that each monograph be comprehensible and of interest to a broad audience. The authors provide an authoritative treatment of important problems in major research areas, in which rapid development of new information requires an integrated and reliable evaluation. The series should therefore prove valuable to advanced college students, graduate students, medical students and house staff, practitioners of medicine, laboratory scientists, and teachers.

ABRAHAM G. OSLER
LEON WEISS

Contents

Preface

Chapter 1   Introduction   1

Immune cytotoxic reactions, 4. Allergic reactions, 4.

Chapter 2   The Classical Complement System   6

Introductory comments, 6. Reaction sequence of the classical system, 10. The target cell, 12. Measurement of C components, 14. Assembly and action of C$\overline{1}$, 14. C4 and C2 as substrates for C$\overline{1}$, 17. Formation of the C3 convertase, C$\overline{42}$, 18. Formation of the C5 convertase, EAC$\overline{423}$, 20. C5 and the terminal component reactions, 22. Mechanism of cytolysis, 26. C inhibitors—regulators of C action, 29. Conglutinin and immunoconglutinin, 30.

Chapter 3   Alternate Complement Pathways   32

Constituents of the properdin system, 34. Activation of the properdin system, 41. Cobra venom activation, 49.

Chapter 4   Complement Fixation   56

The dose-response curve in immune hemolysis, 57. Immunoglobulin class and C fixation, 58. The C-fixing sites on immunoglobulin molecules, 61. The conventional procedures, 65. Micro-C-fixation method, 65. The 5 CH$_{50}$ unit method, 67. Quantitative C fixation, 68. Properties of the immune complex with C-fixing ability, 69. The nature of the antigen as a determinant of C fixation, 72. Antigen assays by C fixation, 73. C$\overline{1}$ fixation and transfer test, 76. Estimation of C3, 79. Immune adherence, 80. Complement fixation by protein A from Staphylococcus aureus, 81.

Chapter 5 Developmental Aspects of the Complement System   85

Ontogeny and biosynthesis, 85.   Phylogeny of the C system, 92.   Metabolism of C components, 94. Genetic aspects, 95.   Alternate pathway dysfunction, 105.

Chapter 6 Complement-mediated Host Defense Mechanisms   107

Bactericidal reactions, 107.   Phagocytosis, 110. Virus neutralization, 116.   C receptors on lymphocytes, 120.   Antibody synthesis, 123.

Chapter 7 Additional Aspects of Complement-mediated Cytotoxiticity   128

Immune hemolysis in vivo, 128.   Hemolysis mediated by C and "autoantibodies," 129.   Hemolysis mediated by C in the apparent absence of antibody (paroxysmal nocturnal hemoglobinuria, PNH), 134. Lysis of nucleated cells by antibody and C, 134. Allograft reactions, 137.   Platelet lysis by C and antibody, 140.   C-dependent platelet lysis by unrelated antigen-antibody systems, 142.

Chapter 8 Complement and Inflammation   149

Anaphylatoxins: formation and characterization, 149. Biologic properties of anaphylatoxins, 152.   Other permeability factors, 158.   Blood coagulation, 159.

Chapter 9 Other Types of Complement-associated Tissue Injury   162

C in anaphylaxis mediated by immunoglobulins other than IgE, 163.   Allergic reactions mediated by IgE, 165.   Immune complex diseases, 166.   Arthus reactions, 167.   Shwartzman phenomenon, 168. Serum sickness, 170.   C as a mediator of tissue injury in viral infections, 171.   Leukemia, 173.   Systemic lupus erythematosus (SLE), 175.   Hypocomplementic glomerulonephritis, 179.   Rheumatoid arthritis, 180.   Enhanced C activity levels, 181.   Nonimmune mechanisms of C activation, 183.

Index   185

There is no human thought that does not demand and expect to be perfected, enriched and modified by subsequent experience and reflection . . .
—Benedetto Croce

Preface

This volume is written for the reader who seeks an introduction to the reputedly complex and multifunctional system of plasma proteins called *complement*. Progress in this area has been so extensive in recent years, and the literature so widely scattered, that it appears timely to bring together the newer developments in a volume intended for the general reader rather than the investigator. The need for a comprehensive rather than intensive treatment of the subject appears all the greater since the available reviews have generally been limited to one, or at most a few, aspects of complement activities.

For more than fifty years after its discovery, the term complement was associated with laborious tests of clinical utility and with a small group of investigators who pursued the elusive nature of this laboratory curiosity. For several decades even the existence of complement as a physical entity was questioned. Others maintained that complement had no important physiological function, since citrated plasma, unlike serum, failed to lyse sensitized erythrocytes, the hemolytic reaction used in complement research. This view gained further credence from the finding that the sera of some healthy individuals, one of them an immunologist, was completely inert in the lytic reaction. A rational basis for these anomalies has since been provided through the efforts of many investigators. Their diversified skills have brought many aspects of complement research to the molecular level and have greatly extended our appreciation of complement as a homeostatic system actively engaged in maintaining normal tissue function through its ability to free the body of infectious agents and neoplastic cells. The association of this protective function with toxic by-products and the recognition of complement as a mediator of inflammation and tissue injury have opened many avenues of investigation.

This monograph summarizes these exciting developments which now have relevance for cell biologists as well as for students of immunopathology. The references cited in each chapter have been selected to acquaint the interested student with some of the original publications which highlight the pertinent topics and hopefully guide him to a more intensive study of this subject.

I acknowledge my profound indebtedness to Dr. Michael Heidelberger in whose laboratory and with the guidance of Dr. Manfred Mayer I was introduced to the study of complement. I am grateful to Dr. Jonathan Singer of the University of California in San Diego for the hospitality afforded me during the writing of this monograph, and to Dr. George K. Hirst, Director of The Public Health Research Institute of the City of New York, who granted me a leave for this undertaking. My thanks also go to Mrs. Yelba Chavez and Mrs. Phyllis Simms who prepared the several revisions and the final manuscript patiently and efficiently, and to Mrs. Harriet S. Waks for the index. Ms. Zita de Schauensee of Prentice-Hall was most helpful in editing the manuscript for publication.

ABRAHAM G. OSLER

New York, N.Y.

Chapter 1

Introduction

Recognition of a complement function has been traced to John Hunter, who noted in 1792 that blood putrified more slowly than other substances. Nearly a century later and following the discovery of bacteria, a number of investigators observed that fresh serum destroyed various micro-organisms. This bactericidal property of serum was attributed to the presence of "alexin" (a protective substance), a term suggested by Buchner. He considered the killing action to be enzymatic since it was heat-labile and most readily demonstrable at body temperature. A major advance emerged from the work of Pfeiffer and Bordet, who showed that the destruction of some microorganisms like *V. cholerae* required specific antibody as well as alexin. Bordet also demonstrated that the activity of an antiserum to erythrocytes, which had lost its hemolytic property after heating to 56° C could be fully restored by the addition of fresh normal rabbit serum containing alexin. The term "complement," which we shall refer to as C, was introduced by Ehrlich and Morgenroth. They found that the lytic function resided in the normal serum since the interaction of the anti-serum with the red cells was independent of and preceded hemolysis by C. Antibody served to detect the antigen and prepare the site for the lytic action of C upon the target cell.

These observations, which were completed shortly after the turn of the century, characterized the basic reaction system whose mechanism has since challenged the ingenuity of many dedicated investigators. From the vantage point of hindsight, we can list five major advances which contributed to the central importance now assigned to complement in biology and medicine. The first was recorded by Heidelberger and his associates, who established the physical identity of the action attributed to C and who developed a quantitative methodology for measuring the lytic reaction. These approaches were extended by Mayer through the use of kinetic analyses which facilitated the isolation of reaction intermediates and led to the "one-hit" theory. This theory postulated that a succession of events at a single site, the union of antibody with a cell surface antigen followed by the C-component reaction sequence, is sufficient to cause cell lysis. The third development arose from the demonstration that *in vivo* activation of the C system was causally associated with inflammation and tissue damage. Another advance quickly followed the application of chromatographic and other physiochemical methods for the isolation of serum proteins. The C components in guinea pig and human serum were isolated by Nelson and by Müller-Eberhard in a state of functional and, in some instances, chemical purity. Most recently, the work of several laboratories led to a renewed interest in the properdin system first described by Pillemer, Lepow, and their associates, with the realization that multiple pathways are available for activating the C system (see Chapter 3).

Each of these developments initiated a burst of interest and activity. At this writing, the list of C functions, some more conclusively demonstrated than others, includes: immune destruction of all the formed elements of the blood, i.e., red cells, leukocytes, and platelets; cytocidal action on gram-negative bacteria, treponemes, and protozoa; enhancement of phagocytosis; acceleration of blood clearance through the process of immune adherence; contraction of smooth muscle; increase in vascular permeability; leukotaxis and mobilization of leukocytes, extrusion of lysosomal enzymes, neutralization of viruses and of toxic lipopolysaccharides; involvement in blood clotting and fibrinolysis; generation of kinins; and possibly, participation in cellular immune processes through the presence of C receptors on lymphocytes. This compendium of C activities is by no means final and indicates the extensive range of phenomena into which C research has led. An important contribution of the early experiments was the realization that the hemolytic action of C was diminished or lost if unheated normal serum was previously exposed to an antigen-antibody aggregate. Thus emerged one of the most characteristic properties of C, the ability to combine with an unrelated immune complex in a reaction which deprives the serum of its lytic ability. This phenomenon, so successfully exploited in the Wassermann test for syphilis, has led many investigators to measure serum C levels in a great variety of disease processes in the hope of extracting a meaningful relationship between the two. An association between elevated or diminished hemolytic potency of the serum or of a single C component and a specific disease has been claimed in more than twenty-five clinical situations. Partly because of the imprecision inherent in some assays, the results have often been difficult to interpret and confusing in the sense that elevated as well as diminished hemolytic titers have been reported for a single clinical entity. The basis for these disparities will emerge in later chapters, but it may be useful at this juncture to identify some of the problems which beset attempts to establish a causal rather than a trivial association between altered C activity and etiologic considerations.

The first difficulty has already been alluded to: the capacity of some of the C components to be bound to a variety of immune aggregates. Until the latter are identified and their relation to the disease process under study is established, the finding of a change in hemolytic potency constitutes but a preliminary guide to further investigation. Moreover, changes in hemolytic activity may be induced by factors other than the immune system underlying the disease process. Prominent examples include the rheumatoid factors and conglutinin whose presence in serum can alter C functions. Certain microbial components such as the endotoxins or lipopolysaccharides of gram-negative bacteria, as well as protein components of some staphylococci and streptococci, are highly reactive with the C system. These compounds can diminish the hemolytic activity of serum without the intervention of specific antibody, so that lowered serum C levels do not reflect the major disease process. The staphylococcus A protein, for example, aggregates IgG through interaction with its Fc fragment, thereby initiating the fixation of C. The tissue injury initiated by this event occurs secondarily to that attributed to the several staphylococcal toxins or the interaction of host antibody with the invading pathogen.

Another pertinent example may be drawn from experimental studies of anaphylaxis. Several investigators have reported that the passive systemic anaphylactic reaction in the guinea pig (injection of antiserum followed within a day or two by an intravenous injection of the specific antigen) is associated with a marked depression of hemolytic C activity. When methods were devised for *in vitro* studies of reaginic allergy, these events were reexamined for the system involving IgE and ragweed pollen antigen. The release of histamine, a chemical mediator in anaphylaxis and reaginic allergy, under these conditions appears indifferent to the quantity of early acting C components (C1, C4, and C2) as well as C3 in the reaction mixtures. Nor have C components or their products been found on mast cell membranes in a manner that could implicate them in the release of vasoactive compounds. As a result, most workers accept the conclusion that a secretory rather than a C-dependent reaction sequence modulates histamine release in the allergic and anaphylactic processes despite the diminution of C levels in the latter.

In the light of these comments, it is difficult to stipulate a generally applicable list of criteria that must be fulfilled in order to implicate the C system as a pathogenetic agent of tissue damage. As shown in later discussions, the assignment of a causal role to C as an effector of tissue damage, in distinction to the side reactions of little consequence to the host, requires knowledge of the fate of individual C components and their cleavage products at the sites of tissue injury and the identification of C-dependent reaction intermediates in intimate association with the pathologic process. In some instances even this evidence is not conclusive. The development of appropriate *in vitro* models has been very helpful in this regard since these allow greater freedom in manipulating the levels of the individual C components and in following the consequences of their alterations in terms of their pathogenetic functions. Studies with these models and the *in vivo* events which they represent have led to the identification of three major pathways of antibody mediated tissue injury associated with specific immunoglobulins. Their major characteristics are summarized in Table 1-1.

IMMUNE CYTOTOXIC REACTIONS

These reactions are mediated only by those immunoglobulins capable of activating the C sequence. The immunoglobulins act by binding specific antigenic determinants on the target cell membrane through their Fab fragments. For the sheep erythrocyte, the antigen involved in the cytolytic process is a glycolipid, the Forssman antigen.

Generally, the immune complex on the cell membrane provides the C activation site in the Fc portion of the antibody. Although exceptions are known which involve the $F(ab')_2$ dimer, C activation by this means does not usually culminate in hemolysis.

Completion of the C reaction sequence on the cell surface leads to irreversible membrane damage.

The tissue damage results from target cell destruction and not because the cell constituents are necessarily toxic.

ALLERGIC REACTIONS

Due to Reaginic Antibodies of the IgE *Class, as in Hay Fever*

These immunoglobulins bind to cell receptors through the Fc portion, a binding unrelated to specific antigenic determinants on the cell surface.

Immune complexes then formed through the union of the Fab fragments with multivalent antigens activate a membrane adenyl cyclase leading to an increase in the intracellular levels of cyclic adenosine monophosphate. Vasoactive compounds like histamine are released from their membrane-bound vesicles without accompanying cell death. The ensuing tissue damage results from the release of pharmacologically active agents such as histamine and serotonin and not necessarily through cell death.

Due to Nonreaginic Immunoglobulins, as in Anaphylaxis due to IgG

The release of histamine and other vasoactive agents can be mediated by immunoglobulins such as the IgG1 in the guinea pig, rabbit, and other species. These antibodies activate the C system through the alternate pathway (see Chapter 3), but C utilization is not necessarily required to elicit the anaphylactic response. Thus, a C requirement has not been demonstrated in local or systemic anaphylactic reactions involving prior antibody fixation. Utilization of C does however lead to the production of highly active C component cleavage products, such as the anaphylatoxins. These peptides are potent inflammatory agents whose properties and modes of action are discussed in Chapter 8. In addition, the destruction of platelets, vascular endothelium, and other tissues through the intervention of preformed immune aggregates is dependent upon C activation.

Table 1–1

| | Cytotoxic reactions | Allergic reactions mediated by: | |
		IgE	IgG
1. Antibody class	IgM, IgG		
2. Mode of cell binding	Through Fab to antigenic determinants on the cell membrane	Through Fc on basophils	Through Fc on basophils and through preformed immune aggregates on platelets
3. C activation	Through hinge region of Fc piece after union with antigen	May occur but appears to be inconsequential	Not considered essential for mediator release from basophils. With platelets as target cells, C activation occurs in the fluid phase leading to binding of complexes and release of mediators
4. C pathway utilized	Classical	Properdin—feebly	Both pathways are triggered but platelet release reaction is primarily due to alternative (properdin) pathway function
5. Fate of cell	Destroyed	Cell remains viable	Basophils remain viable. Platelets are destroyed
6. Released components	Cell contents	Histamine, serotonin, SRS-A, and chemotactic agents	Same as for IgE for basophils. Platelets release vasoactive amines, peptides, and cellular macromolecules

Chapter 2

The Classical Complement System

INTRODUCTORY COMMENTS

Until 1969 the term "complement" was used to describe a system of eleven serum glycoproteins and several inhibitors whose sequential interaction can be initiated by aggregated immunoglobulins. During the past few years it has become increasingly evident that this sequence has important branch points with alternate means of activation. The relative importance of the several pathways for maintaining host viability and the possible interrelationships between the different activation routes are now under active investigation. This chapter is devoted to a description of the classical or conventional pathway which has now been studied for almost a century.

Complement is represented by the letter C. The individual components which comprise the classical system are listed in the order of their interaction and are designated

C1, C4, C2, C3, C5, C6, C7, C8, and C9.

Since C4 was found to react before C2 and C3, the numerical sequence has given way to considerations of reaction mechanisms. The nine components contain eleven proteins because the first component, C1, occurs and acts as a trimolecular complex containing C1q, C1r, and C1s. The physicochemical properties of these constituents in human serum are given in Table 2-1. The classical system also includes several inactivators of individual components which exert a homeostatic function on the C system. They are described in Table 2-2.

Before discussing the reaction sequence involving these components, it should be noted that the criteria of purity upon which the data in Table 2-1 are based were largely derived from electrophoretic, chromatographic, and ultracentrifugal studies. Work on the chemical structure of several components now under way in several laboratories, will clarify their mechanisms of interaction in molecular terms. Application of protein separation techniques to the C system has made available preparations of the individual

6

Table 2-1

Physiochemical properties of proteins in the human classical complement sequence

Recommended * nomenclature		Previous designation	Electrophoretic mobility of human components	Molecular weight	Serum concentration, μg/ml	Relative activity, CH_{50}/ml §	Some cleavage products
C1	C1q	11S component, C'0	γ2	400,000	190	C1-74,000	
	C1r		β	170,000‡	180		
	C1s	C1a † esterase (after activation)	α2	113,000	230		Yields two fragments, of mol. wt. 77,000 and 36,000 after reduction
C4		β1E	β1	204,000	450	12,000	C4a (6,000 daltons) and C4b (198,000 daltons)
C2			β2	117,000	25	2,600	C2a, C2b, C2 kinin
C3		β1C	β1	195,000	1230	20,000	C3a, C3b, C3c, C3d
C5		β1F	β1	185,000	75	1,300	C5a, C5b
C6			β2	95,000	60	3,000	
C7			β2	120,000	65	1,500	
C8			γ1	153,000	< 10	5,000	
C9			α2	79,000	< 10	12,800	

* Based on recommendations approved by the World Health Organization. Bull. Wld. Hlth. Org. **39**:935, 1968.
† The suffix "a" was used to denote the acquisition of enzymatic activity. Currently, a bar is used in place of the suffix "a." Thus the term for the esterase C1a is now C$\bar{1}$.
‡ As estimated by Bing and associates, J. Immunol., **113**:225, 1974.
§ CH_{50} refers to the number of 50% hemolytic units. The actual numbers will vary with different titration procedures.

Table 2–2

Inhibitors of complement component interactions

Factor	Abbreviation or synonym	Molecular weight	Activity
C$\bar{1}$ inactivator	C$\bar{1}$INH	90,000	Inactivates lytic and enzymatic effects of C$\bar{1}$ fixed or in free solution; also inhibits kallikrein, plasmin, and Hageman factor; an α2 neuraminoglycoprotein.
C3b inactivator	KAF; C3 INA	100,000	Reacts with fixed C3b, thereby interfering with immune lysis, adherence, and phagocytosis. Renders bound C3 sensitive to trypsin.
C4 inactivator			Isolated by Jensen from nurse shark serum; utilizes human C4 and Na-tosyl-L-arginine methyl ester as substrates.
C4b inactivator			A β-1 globulin isolated by Cooper.
C6 inactivator			Inactivates the intermediate EAC142356.

components which are functionally pure, i.e., they provide only a single component activity. These, in turn, have been used to prepare potent antisera which have been helpful in monitoring the quantity and fate of the individual C components in sera and other body fluids and tissues. The components in human sera, and some of the guinea pig reagents as well as their antisera, are now available commercially. Some of these preparations may contain other serum constituents as minor contaminants. Purification of the C components and knowledge of their physicochemical properties have provided the basis for critical and definitive mechanistic studies. For example, it is now possible to measure C component interaction in terms of specific activities, i.e., ratios of hemolytic to weight units.

The term "hemolytic activity" does not take into account the side reactions which occur on the cell membrane and in the fluid phase of reaction mixtures. These events do not participate in the destruction of the target cell and may, in fact, impede its progress. These considerations gave rise to the expression "effective molecules," a critical concept in terms of understanding the hemolytic reaction as applied to the interaction of individual components. The dissection of the reaction sequence was greatly facilitated by the elaboration of Mayer's "one-hit" theory which will be discussed later as it applies to immune hemolysis.

These fundamental achievements which ushered in the modern approaches to C research had their origins in two earlier developments, namely, the recognition of C as a multicomponent system and the utilization of quantitative procedures for measuring the extent of hemolysis. The former was initiated in 1907 by Ferrata, who pursued the earlier finding of Buchner that dialysis of fresh guinea pig serum against water yielded a precipitate and a hemolytically inert supernatant fluid. Ferrata was able to restore lysis by recombining the dissolved precipitate with the supernatant. The factors in the precipitate were named "midpiece" by Brand, who noted that the combination of this fraction with the antibody-coated red cells (sensitized cells) was essential for the subsequent action of the supernatant in the hemolytic sequence. He named the activity of the latter "endpiece." These experiments demonstrated the sequential nature of C action and laid the basis for studies of the reaction intermediates on the sensitized cell surface. Evidence for a third component emerged from experiments with guinea pig serum that had been inactivated by treatment with either cobra venom or yeast cells. In 1926 a fourth component was found in serum rendered hemolytically inert by treatment with ammonia and other primary amines. The sequence of action of these four components was clarified by Ueno in 1938, and characterization of these reagents was begun by Pillemer in 1941. During these years, the mechanism of antibody-mediated lysis by C was studied with the "R" reagents, serum preparations presumably devoid of one component but containing an excess of the remaining three. Many of these experiments were difficult to interpret. The R reagents were not functionally homogeneous, so it was often difficult to characterize the intermediates in the sequence or to identify the component which limited the reaction. An additional difficulty during this period was the lack of a precise method for estimating the extent of hemolysis. This obstacle was overcome by the development in 1946 of a quantitative spectrophotometric procedure for the titration of C based on the use of a 50% hemolytic endpoint, the CH_{50} unit, as the basis of measurement.

The introduction of a quantitative methodology for the study of immune hemolysis led to a critical appraisal of the many parameters which influence the course of this reaction. These include the reaction temperature, electrolyte concentration, red cell number, pH, volume, the nature, and the amount of antibody used in sensitizing the erythrocytes. The spectrophotometric analyses also facilitated the demonstration that calcium and magnesium were essential cofactors in immune hemolysis, thereby setting the stage for characterizing the reaction intermediates by means of kinetic studies as a basis for formulating the single-hit hypothesis. This concept departed from previous theories which held that the sigmoid dose-response relationships of lysis by C was due to cell heterogeneity or cumulative damage to the erythrocyte membrane. These interpretations were abandoned when Mayer and his colleagues demonstrated that a plot of the degree of lysis as a function of individual component concentration ($C\overline{1}$, C4, C2, or C9) yielded curves which rose from the origin and were entirely concave to the abscissa.

The quantitative treatment of the noncumulative, one-hit hypothesis was achieved through application of the Poisson distribution function, based on the likelihood that a single lesion may lead to lysis under appropriate conditions. This relationship is expressed as $z = -\ln(1 - y)$, where z equals the average number of hits per cell and y is the fraction of cells lysed. When $z = 1$, the value of y is 0.63, indicating that 63% of the cells have been destroyed when the average number of lesions per cell is unity. Given the cell number and optimal experimental conditions, the titration of individual components in terms of "effective molecules" is thus readily achieved for mechanistic studies. With components of adequate purity, these assays combined with weight analyses have yielded valuable information regarding the efficiency of a component in the hemolytic sequence, the stability of reaction intermediates, and the stoichiometry of component interaction needed to lyse the target cell by antibody and C. The accumulated evidence has overwhelmingly supported the theory that immune cytolysis is a one-hit, noncumulative process.

REACTION SEQUENCE OF THE CLASSICAL SYSTEM

The Antibody

Studies of immune hemolysis have generally employed the system comprising sheep erythrocytes, rabbit antiserum to the Forssman antigen, and guinea pig C. The Forssman antigen is a membrane glycolipid present in sheep erythrocytes and in many other cell types. Customarily, rabbits are immunized with boiled sheep erythrocyte stromata to obtain immune sera rich in hemolytic antibodies predominantly of the IgM class. The latter are particularly useful because of their potent hemolytic capacity. The heterogeneity of different immunoglobulin classes in terms of their lytic potential, i.e., their ability to activate the C sequence, is not limited to rabbit antisera. The electrophoretically rapid IgGl guinea pig immunoglobulins are virtually inert with respect to the classical C sequence, as compared to the IgG2 immunoglobulins present in the same serum sample. An IgG2a mouse myeloma protein did not activate C, but the IgG and IgM classes are efficient in this regard. There are studies with human immunoglobulins which reveal extensive differences in C activation by the several classes and subclasses, as shown in Table 2-3. Human myeloma proteins of the IgG1 and IgG3 subclasses are more active than those of the IgG2 subtype. The IgG4 and IgA immunoglobulins are entirely devoid of hemolytic activity with respect to the classical system. Returning to the Forssman system, it has been estimated that each sheep erythrocyte contains as many as 6×10^5 antibody-binding sites, but this

Table 2–3

Human immunoglobulin class *

	IgG1	IgG2	IgG3	IgG4	IgA1	IgA2	IgM	IgD	IgE
Serum concentration mg/ml	5–12	2–6	0.5–1	0.2–1	0.5–2	0–0.2	0.5–1.5	0–0.4	0.01–0.5
Half-life, days	23	23	16	23	6	6	5	3	2
Placental transfer	+	+	+	+	−	−	−	−	−
Classical C activation †	++	+	++	−	−	−	+	−	−

* From H. L. Spiegelberg, *Advances in Immunology,* 19:265, 1974.
† These studies are based on the use of myeloma proteins.

number provides no information as to the topographical distribution of the antigenic determinants. For the rabbit IgM antibody, this distribution may be of little consequence since Borsos and Rapp have shown that only a single IgM molecule is sufficient to trigger the hemolytic reaction. Through the use of specific activity ratios, they calculated that hemolysis could be initiated when the proportion of antibody to $C\overline{1}$ molecules was unity. For IgG molecules, on the other hand, the ratio was slightly greater than two. The reasonable deduction was made that the antibody molecules unite randomly with the antigenic determinants on the membrane. With the IgM pentamer with as many as ten combining groups for antigen, a single molecule could activate C1 at any membrane site. Twice that number was required for the IgG antibodies. When two IgG molecules were bound in sufficiently close approximation, this "doublet" could then activate the hemolytic system. To achieve a single activated site, it has been calculated that as many as 800 bound molecules of IgG are needed. A rather unique IgG has been described which mimics IgM in its hemolytic behavior, possibly because of its presence in a polymerized form. Human sera apparently contain two subclasses of IgM, only one of which fixes C.

The heightened efficiency of IgM in activating the classical system, long known to workers in this field, can be explained in terms of the relative binding of IgM and IgG for C1q, one of three subcomponents of C1. Bing has established values for these constants through inhibition studies of ^{125}I-labeled C1q binding to an immunosorbent containing covalently bound IgM or other immunoglobulins. The binding constants reported by Bing are 6.42×10^{-6} M for IgM and 1.10×10^{-4} M for IgG. Thus binding of C1q by IgM is more than 500 times greater than by IgG. These values are of the same magnitude as those obtained by different procedures.

THE TARGET CELL

As is well known, antibody-mediated lysis by C may involve cells other than erythrocytes. Rabbit platelets, nucleated cells of many species, gram-negative bacteria, and protozona are all susceptible to destruction by C in the presence of specific antibody which directs the C components to the site of action. The structure of the membrane is, however, a prime determinant for the eventual fate of the cell which has bound a C-fixing immunoglobulin. In bacteria, the gram-negative species undergo irreversible membrane damage leading to cell death. The gram-positive organisms remain viable in the presence of antibody and C until phagocytosis intervenes. This process is followed by intracellular digestion in some instances and multiplication in others. Among erythrocytes of various species, the relative resistance of human red cells to lysis by antibody and C has often been noted. Although the disposition of antigenic determinants on the cell surface may account in part for this insusceptibility, other structural differences must also be considered.. Human red cells are more readily lysed after exposure to proteolytic enzymes, and their membranes have a different net charge than sheep erythrocytes as judged by electrophoretic studies. Unlike the latter, human erythrocytes participate in the immune adherence phenomenon involving antibody and the early C components through C3 (see Chapter 4).

In addition to the properties of the membrane, the antibody and C sources are important factors which govern target cell destruction. The range of this variability for human erythrocytes is indicated in Table 2-4.

Table 2—4

Reactivity of antibodies from different species with different sources of complement *

Complement source	Antibody source				
	Rabbit	G. pig	Dog	Cat	Chicken
Rabbit	200	665	400	250	0
Guinea pig	400	1000	40	65	0
Pig	25	40	65	65	14
Sheep	20	20			
Ox	25	25	25	20	0
Rat	100	100		0	0
Goat	400	400	1000	200	0
Chicken	0	100	20	14	33
Cat	400	400	40	1000	0
Dog	200	200	40	27	0

* From I. Gigli and K. F. Austen, Ann. Rev. Microbiol., 25:309, 1971.

Extensive studies with antisera and C from various mammalian species were carried out by Christine Rice and have been reviewed by Gigli and Austen. It is readily apparent that lysis of these cells is markedly influenced by the source of both the antibody and C. Although these data describe some interesting interrelationships, a critical evaluation would require assurance that the hemolytic systems had been rigorously standardized with respect to such factors as: (a) prior absorption of the C with target cells to remove naturally occurring hemolytic antibodies, (b) the ratio of hemolytic and nonhemolytic immunoglobulins (e.g., IgG1 and IgG2 in the guinea pig) in the antiserum, (c) the divalent cation requirements of the different hemolytic systems, (d) the use of optimal antibody levels for sensitizing the erythrocytes, and (e) the possible participation of alternate pathways. Despite these considerations, the data in Table 2-4 serve as a useful guide to future studies of comparative immunology.

Little attention has been directed in this discussion to the structure and properties of the antibody which prepares the cell for lysis by C, a subject reserved for Chapter 4. The fact that these immunoglobulins only direct the attack by C is indicated by the finding that antibody is dispensable for cell lysis by C. These experiments, first performed several decades ago, have been extended in recent years by McVickar and by Cowan. Reagents such as silicic acid, tannic acid, dextran, polyethylene glycol (Carbowax 4000), and polyvinylpyrrolidone can replace antibody in preparing unsensitized erythrocytes for lysis by C. Relatively high concentrations of these sensitizers are required, e.g., 2 to 6% of Carbowax. These compounds form a readily dissociable complex with cell membrane constituents and mediate lysis in the presence of calcium and the C components. It is thought that these agents induce conformational changes in the membrane which create sites for the activation of C1 and completion of the sequential component reactions. It would be of some interest to ascertain whether an alternate C pathway may also be set into motion by these nonimmune red cell sensitizers.

It has often been observed that marked differences in hemolytic C titrations follow the use of red cells from different sheep. Bell and his colleagues have offered an explanation which probably accounts for many of the observed differences. Titrations were performed with a single preparation of rabbit hemolysin and human C, but with cells of three types from different sheep. The sheep were classified in terms of the K^+ content of their erythrocytes and their antigenic determinants as follows: low or high K^+ and antigenic types LL, LM, and MM. The evidence accumulated by these investigators and earlier by De Bracco and Dalmasso showed that the lytic susceptibility of the cells to C and antibody decreased as follows: $LK^+(LL) > LK^+(LM) > HK^+(MM)$. Substitution of an IgG hemolysin for IgM did not alter the susceptibility to immune lysis which varied with the intracellular K^+ levels from 17 to 49 to 76% lysis for cells with low, medium, and high K^+. Genetic factors also contributed to this variability since cells of the $LK^+(LL)$ type were lysed more readily than those of the $LK^+(LM)$ type. When K^+ was substituted for Na^+ in the buffer diluent used in the titrations, the CH_{50} titers were reduced in half with HK^+ cells. The LK^+ cells were less affected by the extracellular K^+ levels. From a practical viewpoint, the use of pooled sheep erythrocytes tends to minimize these differences and is recommended for general use.

MEASUREMENT OF C COMPONENTS

The nine components and eleven C proteins can be estimated in several ways. These include use of the R reagents, the method based on cellular intermediates, enzymatic techniques, and immunodiffusion. As already mentioned, the use of the R reagents was based on the assumption that the reagent in question was multifunctional, lacking only the specific component under study. In addition to the relative insensitivity of this procedure, neither of the two assumptions could withstand rigorous experimental verification; so these procedures have been largely discontinued. Studies based on the characterization of the cellular intermediates have been far more rewarding in terms of delineating the mechanism of interaction of the nine components and the stoichiometry of their activities. The results obtained by these procedures enabled the description of C action in molecular terms and are summarized in the sections which follow. The enzymatic approach, as shown below, is applicable only to several of the intermediates found during the sequential component interaction. These are serum proteases which exert limited fragmentation of the next component in the sequence, e.g., C2, C4, C3, and C5, with the liberation of low molecular weight peptides, some of which possess potent biological activity. Immunodiffusion and immunoelectrophoretic analyses provide additional characterization of the components and their fragments and identify their antigenic composition. In addition, the use of radial immunodiffusion with monospecific antisera offers one means of immunochemical quantitation.

ASSEMBLY AND ACTION OF $C\overline{1}$

Our knowledge regarding the sequence of component interactions on a molecular basis is derived from kinetic studies with purified reactants and application of the one-hit theory. Estimation of the capacity of a given component to participate in the activation, binding, assembly, and conversion to an active intermediate, a sequence that permits its titration on a molecular basis, is predicated on the availability of an excess of the appropriate receptors. In addition, experimental conditions must be adjusted to assure an excess of all other components so that both the rate and extent of lysis will be governed only by the activity of the component under study. Completion of the sequence is regulated by control mechanisms which include inhibitors of several of the activated components and the rapid decay of a few intermediates as discussed below.

The interaction of the first C component with an immune complex in solution or on the surface of a sensitized erythrocyte (EA) typifies important aspects of this sequential reaction mechanism. These include the existence in serum of inert precursors, their assembly through the appearance of binding sites on the prior intermediate, and enzymatic attack on the next component in the reaction chain. For C1, the physiologic stimulus is an immune complex composed of multivalent antigen or cell surface determinants bound to multivalent antibody. As noted, there are thousands of antigenic sites on the erythrocyte. Their union with antibody is designated by the term EA. With respect to the lytic mechanism however, the critical events are those that occur on a single site, S. In accord with the one-hit hypothesis, the sequential reactions at one site which result in the construction of a complex involving all nine components are sufficient and necessary for cell lysis.

$C\bar{1}$ is the first enzyme to be formed in the C sequence. As shown by Lepow, the inactive precursor is found in human serum as a calcium-dependent trimolecular complex. In the absence of calcium or in the presence of a chelating agent like ethylenediaminetetraacetate, the trimer dissociates into its three components called C1q, C1r, and C1s. Recombination of the three subunits in the presence of calcium into a complex with the molecular composition of $C1q_1r_2s_4$ is essential for the expression of its enzymatic and hemolytic properties.

The properties of C1q (originally called the 11S or C'O component) are of considerable interest. This molecule possesses the recognition site for antibody and is unusual because of its resemblance to a collagen-like glycoprotein containing hydroxyproline and hydroxylysine with a lysine content approximating 18% of all amino acids. Ultrastructural studies by Polley and by Stroud and their associates indicate that C1q is an extremely fragile molecule containing three morphologically distinctive parts which have been visualized in the electron microscope. A central subunit is connected to six terminal units by means of six thin strands. Presumably, these terminal units account for the multiple combining groups on the C1q molecule for the immunoglobulins. Porter's recent studies indicate that each of the six C1q subunits consists of three polypeptide chains which form a triple helix, and their globular ends provide the binding sites for the immunoglobulin. Bing has suggested that anionic and hydrophobic residues in the C1q molecule participate in binding immunoglobulins. The microscopic studies also suggest that C1q exists as a disc-like coil capable of unfolding to a rod-like structure. The binding of C1q to the Fc portions of certain immunoglobulins leads to the formation of three-dimensional aggregates which form visible precipitables at sufficiently high concentrations. This process may therefore serve as an amplification mechanism for additional C1q-antibody complexes. The binding of C1q to immune aggregates has been exploited in a relatively simple purification procedure.

C1r has recently been isolated as a homogeneous protein and, although some of its physicochemical properties have been described, its mode of interaction with C1q is not yet clear. It is thought that the union of C1q with C1r induces a conformational change in the former which facilitates the binding of C1s and its conversion to the catalytic state, $\overline{C1s}$. This conversion may also occur after C1s has been subjected to the action of plasmin or trypsin. $\overline{C1s}$ contains two major subunits whose combined molecular weight is 113,000 daltons. It has been known for some time that the compound di-isopropylfluorophosphate (DFP) inhibited the action of $\overline{C1}$ in the lytic sequence, and it was on the basis of this finding by Lepow, Levine, and Becker that the esterase nature of $\overline{C1}$ was established. The catalytic site on C1 is located on the C1s subunit which cannot bind to an immune complex in the absence of C1q and C1r. The binding site of DFP has now been localized to a polypeptide chain of 36,000 daltons in the activated $\overline{C1s}$ molecule. These experiments have made it abundantly clear that C1 exists in serum as a proenzyme that is activated in the sequence outlined above. The esterolytic nature of $\overline{C1}$ also became evident when it was shown to hydrolyse certain synthetic substrates such as p-toluenesulfonyl-L-arginine methyl ester, TAME, and N-acetyl tyrosine ethyl ester (ATE), and that this activity paralleled its capacity to support immune hemolysis. Inhibition of $\overline{C1}$ activity by DFP and other phosphonate esters led Becker and Austen to suggest that the $\overline{C1}$ esterase resembles trypsin. It has been further suggested that a serine residue is present in the catalytic site which is localized to a different portion of the molecule than its binding site for antibody. This conclusion is also derived from experiments with the inhibitor carageenan, a high molecular weight polysaccharide that inhibits the hemolytic but not the enzymatic function of $\overline{C1}$. Bing, Cory and others demonstrated that compounds containing substituted benzamidine or sulfonyl fluoride groups are potent inhibitors of $\overline{C1}$ at levels of 10^{-6} to 10^{-5} M.

Several other inhibitors of $\overline{C1}$ have been identified, but the naturally occurring serum protein called $\overline{C1}$INH is by far the most important. Its homeostatic role is considered in the discussion of hereditary angioedema (see Chapter 5). This inhibitor has been found in guinea pig and human serum and prevents the hemolytic as well as enzymatic functions of $C\bar{1}$.

Heidelberger postulated that the macromolecular complex, C1, forms a loose and dissociable union with gamma globulin which is intensified when it binds to immune complexes. In an extension of these studies, Borsos showed that the hemolytic efficiency of $C\bar{1}$ is markedly affected by the ionic strength of the reaction medium, being greatly enhanced at lower values, with optimal binding at $\mu = 0.065$. Reversible inactivation occurs upon restoration to isotonic levels, and these activity changes can be correlated with alterations in the sedimentation constants of C1 and $C\bar{1}$. These interesting findings have been used in the design of an exquisitely sensitive $C\bar{1}$ fixation assay which has had important applications in defining the molecular composition of reaction intermediates (see Chapter 4).

It may be noted in passing that a variety of compounds other than aggregated immunoglobulins interact with C1. These include RNA, DNA, several polynucleotides, sulfated polysaccharides, and enzymes such as trypsin, plasmin, and those present in mammalian lysosomes.

C4 AND C2 AS SUBSTRATES FOR $C\bar{1}$

Unlike C1q which binds to an immunoglobulin site in an immune aggregate without prior activation, the addition of C4 and C2 to the $EAC\bar{1}$ site is preceded by an activation step involving proteolytic cleavage by the enzyme formed in the previous reaction step. Like C1, the component C4 is present in serum in an inert form. Studies in Müller-Eberhard's laboratory indicate that C4 is composed of three polypeptide chains with molecular weights of 87,000, 78,000, and 33,000 daltons. When subjected to the action of $C1\bar{s}$, the α chain (87,000 mol. wt.) is cleaved, liberating a peptide of 6000 daltons and exposing a labile-binding site for the further participation of C4 in immune hemolysis. Upon interaction with cell-bound $C\bar{1}$, i.e., $EAC\bar{1}$, C4 (mol. wt. = 204,000) undergoes proteolytic cleavage, a highly labile binding site is exposed, and the intermediate $EAC\bar{1}4b$ is formed with the release of a small fragment, C4a. The presence of an activation step was deduced by Cooper and Müller-Eberhard. They observed that only about 20% of the available C4 molecules were capable of binding to the sensitized erythrocyte because of the transitory nature of the binding site. Unless the activated molecules containing the binding sites collided with cell-bound $C\bar{1}$, they became incapable of furthering immune hemolysis. Another problem arose when it was shown that only a small percentage of the cell-bound C4 molecules was hemolytically active. The paucity of $EAC\bar{1}4$ sites capable of hemolytically fruitful reactions instigated a search for other sites containing

C4. At least three others have been described by Borsos and Rapp. One of these can combine with the next component in the series, C2, without going on to lysis, possibly because of rapid decay. A second site may become hemolytically functional with a further increment of antiserum that may provide an additional source of the later, heat-stable components. The third site that contains C4 may be detected with a monospecific anti-serum to C4—but this site cannot be converted to a hemolytically active form.

The hemolytic progression involving $EAC\bar{1}$ and C4 may be written as

$$EAC\bar{1} + C4 \longrightarrow EAC\bar{1}4b + 4a$$

where 4a is the minor cleavage fragment with a molecular weight of 6000 daltons.

It is thus apparent that the consumption of C4 proceeds simultaneously on the cell membrane site containing $EAC\bar{1}$ and in the fluid phase. In the former instance, the interaction with the other C components may lead to lysis, but the extent of this terminal event will depend on such factors as sensitized cell concentration, the availability of C4, as well as the rate of the competing fluid phase destruction of C4. Like several of the other components (C2, C3, and C5) C4 is very sensitive to tryptic digestion, a susceptibility which may be related to its ease of activation in the hemolytic system as well as to the ease of its degradation in the fluid phase.

The reactions discussed thus far can be written schematically as:

$$E + A \rightarrow EA + C1q + C1r + C1s \xrightarrow{\text{Ca}^{++}} EAC\bar{1} \quad + \quad C4 \longrightarrow EAC14b + C4a$$

$$\downarrow + C\bar{1}\ \text{INH} \qquad \downarrow + C\bar{1}$$

$$\text{Inactive} \qquad C4a + C4b$$
$$\text{complex}$$

FORMATION OF THE C3 CONVERTASE, $\overline{C42}$

The entry of C2 into this sequence requires Mg^{2+} and constitutes the final step in the assembly of the proteolytic enzyme $\overline{C42}$, whose natural substrate is C3. The molecular weight of this enzyme called the C3 con-vertase, has been estimated at 300,000 daltons. In addition to C3 this enzyme can utilize acetyl glycine methyl ester as substrate. It may be noted that $\overline{C42}$ can exert its catalytic action after $C\bar{1}$ has been removed from the intermediate EAC142 by the action of a chelating agent. The interaction with C2 parallels the steps involving C4 in that $C\bar{1}$ can also cleave C2 in the fluid phase, in a reaction that reduces the hemolytic efficiency of this component. Thus we have the addition of the major cleavage fragment C2a to the cellular intermediate as well as cleavage of C2 in the fluid phase. $C\overline{1}$ alone splits C2, but the rate of this reaction is accelerated in the presence of C4.

$$EAC\overline{1} + C2 \xrightarrow{Mg^{++}} C2a + C2b \text{ (low molecular weight}$$
$$\text{degradation product)}$$

$$EAC\overline{1}4b + C2a \longrightarrow EAC\overline{142} \text{ or } EAC\overline{42}$$

The molecular weight of C2b has been estimated at 34,000 daltons, but this fragment has not yet been isolated, possibly because of further degradation by $C\overline{1}$ or other serum enzymes. Mayer has pointed out that the adsorption of C2 is very rapid even at low temperatures, while the formation of the hemolytically active complex proceeds much more slowly. The final product of this assembly, $EAC\overline{42}$ is unstable at 37° C and undergoes fairly rapid decay unless there is a sufficient quantity of C3 in the vicinity of the cell-bound complex to mediate the next step in the sequence. The decayed product is hemolytically inactive. Again, in parallelism to the situation with C4, only a minute proportion of the C2 molecules is detectable by hemolytic measurements with guinea pig serum, although the number can be greatly increased by substituting rat serum as a source of the late-acting components. When purified components are used, the hemolytic efficiency of C2 can be shown to approximate 100%.

Once the active intermediate containing C2 has been formed, $C\overline{1}$ is dispensable. This fact has been used in the design of the $C\overline{1}$ fixation and transfer test, noted above and described in Chapter 4, which is based on the discovery that a quantitative transfer of $C\overline{1}$ can be effected from various immune complexes to EAC4 by raising the ionic strength from $\mu = 0.065$ to $\mu = 0.15$. There is some evidence that C4 and C2 exist as a loose, readily dissociable complex until acted upon by the $C1\overline{s}$ esterase. Treatment of human but not of guinea pig C2 with iodine enhances its reactivity some 20-fold by retarding decay of the $EAC\overline{42}$ intermediate.

Recent developments in our understanding of C4 and C2 involvement have emerged from the studies by Rapp and Borsos and their colleagues. These investigators found that sensitized erythrocytes which had bound $C\overline{1}$ and C4, i.e., $EAC\overline{1}4$, were more susceptible to lysis by rat C-EDTA (rat serum containing the chelating agent EDTA) than by guinea pig C-EDTA regardless of the amount of C2 that was added to further the hemolytic sequence. As originally noted by Miyakawa and others, the American workers were able to effect a 25-fold increase in human C4 and C2 activities through the use of rat C-EDTA as a converting agent. From kinetic and endpoint experiments designed to limit the amounts of C1, C4, or C2 for preparing the intermediate $EAC\overline{1}42$, they deduced that with limited C1, clusters of $C\overline{42}$ are formed in the vicinity of a single site containing C1. In addition, as noted previously, numerous C4 molecules, probably C4b, are attached to the cell membrane. Only some of the $C\overline{42}$ complexes can be lysed with guinea pig C-EDTA, but 100% of these sites are reactive with rat C-EDTA. Use of the latter reagent which renders every $C\overline{42}$ site hemolytically productive led to the estimates of the number of molecules of C1, C4, and C2 in guinea pig and human sera shown in Table 2-5.

Table 2–5

	Guinea pig serum	Human serum
	No. molecules per ml	
C1	8.8×10^{12}	3.8×10^{13}
C4	1.8×10^{14}	2×10^{14}
C2	1.1×10^{14}	3.1×10^{12} *

* After oxidation, this number is increased 2.6×10^{13}. (From T. Borsos et al., *5th Int'l Symp. of the Canadian Soc. for Immunol.*, S. Karger, Basel, 1970, p. 27.)

The tryptic-like action of $C\overline{1}$ has been demonstrated in experiments showing that admixture of human or guinea pig C2 with trypsin in the presence of $EAC\overline{14}$ forms a converting enzyme which is indistinguishable from that formed by the action of $C\overline{1}$.

The assembly and activation of $EAC\overline{42}$ is of singular importance. As discussed in the preceding section, this enzyme results from a complex series of events involving assembly and activation of $C\overline{1}$, cleavage of C4 and C2, binding and assembly of the larger fragments, loss of C1, and finally, rearrangement to form a new enzyme whose natural substrate is the complement protein C3. As shown in Table 2-1, C3 is by far the major C component in serum on a weight basis, comprising as it does more than half of all the complement proteins. Human serum contains more than 1 mg of C3 per ml. Electron microscopic studies by Suzuki and collaborators indicate that the molecule of C3 appears to be roughly spherical with a rugged perimeter and is composed of eighteen spherical elements, each of molecular weight approximating 10,000 daltons. Müller-Eberhard has reported that C3 is composed of two polypeptide chains with a combined molecular weight of 195,000 daltons.

FORMATION OF THE C5 CONVERTASE, $EAC\overline{423}$

With respect to the classical sequence, the complex $C\overline{42}$ cleaves C3, exposing a binding site on the major fragment, C3b, which as shown by Shin forms a new intermediate $EAC\overline{423}$ that is proteolytic for C5, the next component in the sequence. EAC$\overline{423}$, like its predecessor EAC$\overline{42}$, may decay into an inactive form through the loss of C2. However its half-life, when prepared with oxidized C2, is about 3 hr at 37° C. The limited proteolysis of C3 marks a reaction step which occurs in both the classical and alternate pathways through the mediation of different enzymes. This reaction step is of central importance since it initiates the production of intermediates and by-products for many of the biologic functions of C.

The interaction of EAC$\overline{42}$ with C3 can be depicted as follows:

$$EAC\overline{42} + C3 \longrightarrow EAC\overline{423}b + C3a$$

The C3 fragment which forms the intermediate EAC$\overline{423}$ is called C$\overset{*}{3}$b. It is the major portion of the C3 molecule whose molecular weight is 185,000. The molecular weight of C3a is about 9000 daltons. C3b not only provides the link between the classical and alternate pathways (see Chapter 3) but also enables immune complexes to participate in immune adherence reactions (see Chapter 4). The biologic activity of the EAC$\overline{423}$b intermediate is normally regulated by the inhibitor C3INA. Cell-bound C3b may also undergo limited proteolysis to release the fragment C3c and retain C3d on the membrane. These two fragments can be distinguished through their antigenic properties. Treatment of purified C3 with trypsin also yields the fragments C3a, C3b, and C3c.

The data in Fig. 2-1 summarize the results of an experiment in which the number of EAC$\overline{423}$ sites formed per cell is plotted as a function of

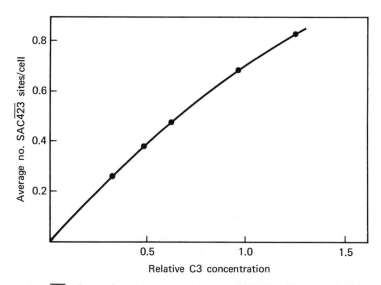

Fig. 2-1. SAC $\overline{423}$ refers to the total number of hemolytically active sites in the entire cell population. (From H. S. Shin and M. M. Mayer, *Biochemistry,* **7**: 3001, 1968.)

the relative C3 concentration. The ordinate scale is expressed in terms of Z or $-\ln(1-y)$ to illustrate an application of the Poisson function in the study of C component interactions at the molecular level. Given a highly purified preparation of C3, of known molecular weight, it is thus possible to calculate the number of C3 molecules added to attain a given level of Z and estimate the efficiency of $EAC\overline{423}$ formation.

C5 AND THE TERMINAL COMPONENT REACTIONS

The entry of C5 into the reaction sequence has been viewed somewhat differently by various investigators. Some proposed that C5, C6, and C7 act only by combining to form a functional trimolecular complex somewhat analogous to C1q,r,s. Others believed that, like its predecessors, C5 also acts individually, coming into play after formation of the complex $EAC\overline{423}$.

Recent experiments by Arroyave, Kolb, and Müller-Eberhard with the human components C5 through C9 have largely resolved this issue. In the fluid phase of reaction mixtures, reversible interaction was observed between C5 and C6 in the absence of C7, and between C5 and C7 in the absence of C6. When a reaction mixture was prepared with all three of the components, enhanced association of C5, C6, and C7 resulted in the formation of the trimolecular complex, C5,6,7.

A slightly different and more complex series of events occurred between $EAC\overline{4,2,3}$ and the purified components. The $C\overline{423}$ enzyme yielded a stable complex with C5 and C6 as had been previously noted with guinea pig reagents by Mayer and his associates. This complex was capable of binding to $EAC\overline{423}$ in the presence of C7 to form the hemolytically competent EAC423567. Moreover, the C5,6 complex could also be attached to nonsensitized red cells, E, in the presence of C7. Trypsin and plasmin also generate these complexes so that both $EAC\overline{4,2,3}$ and $EC\overline{4,2,3}$ can then bind C5,6 in the presence of C7 and proceed to lysis upon the addition of C8 and C9. The lysis of E under these conditions, in the absence of antibody, has been termed "reactive lysis." Mayer and others have recently identified another intermediate called pseudo-EAC6 which lacks C2a but is lysed in the presence of activated C5. Reactive lysis is less efficient than the immune, antibody-dependent process, since the complexes which mediate this reaction are short-lived until they bind to the receptors on E. In the absence of antibody-directed sites of action, the complexes soon become inactive. In addition to the action on E and EA by C5,6,7, some nucleated mammalian cells, gram-negative bacteria and liposomes also become susceptible to lysis by this trimolecular complex upon the addition of C8 and C9.

The affinity between C5, C6, and C7 in free solution and the equimolarity of the cell-bound equivalents strongly support the concept of a firm trimolecular assembly on the cell membrane as a basis for the final attack by C8 and C9. This trimolecular complex forms only in the simultaneous presence of C5, C6, and C7.

The fate of C5 in these events is known. This component undergoes limited proteolysis by $EAC\overline{4,2,3}$ to yield a major fragment, 5b, with a molecular weight of 164,000 and a binding site for the C5-cleaving enzyme to form the next intermediate in the sequence, $EAC\overline{4,2,3},5$. This product is thermolabile in the absence of C6 and C7. The thermolability of $EAC\overline{4,2,3},5$ and $EAC\overline{42}$ intermediates suggests that these are the rate-limiting steps in the sequence ultimately leading to cell lysis. The cell-bound C5b remains firmly attached, though inactive when decayed. The minor cleavage fragment of C5, called C5a, like C3 has anaphylatoxic properties. The synthetic ester, N-acetyl-L-tryosylethylester, a competitive peptidase inhibitor, blocks cleavage of C5 and the formation of the $EAC\overline{4,2,3},5$ intermediate. Proteolytic cleavage of C5 can also be effected by trypsin, plasmin, and lysosomal enzymes. Electron microscopic studies of sensitized erythrocytes subjected to the sequential addition of C components revealed ultrastructural lesions on cells which have bound C1, C4, C2, C3 and C5. The number of these lesions correlated favorably with the number of C5 molecules added to form this intermediate. These membrane alterations are not functional since they do not lead to permeability defects, and their number remains fairly constant even when the sequence is completed with all nine components.

The assembly of the complex which completes the sequence and which represents the attack mechanism on cell membranes has also been elucidated in Müller-Eberhard's laboratory and is depicted in Fig. 2-2. These workers studied the association of the purified components C5, C6, C7, C8, and C9 as isolated proteins and in serum with the aid of sucrose density gradients. Reversible complexes were observed between the following components: C5 + C6; C5 + C7; C5 + C6 + C7; C5 + C8; C5 + C6 + C7 + C8; C8 + C9; and C5 + C7 + C8 + C9. These findings, like those discussed above, attest to the formation of the trimolecular complex C5,6,7 and demonstrate a single binding site between this complex and C8. The C8 now bound in a tetramolecular complex, furnished binding sites for six C9 molecules to complete the final attack mechanism, i.e., a reversible complex composed of C5,6,7,8,9 with a sedimentation constant of 22.5S and a molecular weight approaching 10^6 daltons. A curious aspect of this complex is the apparent assembly of six C9 molecules as compared to single molecules of the other four components in the decamolecular cytolytic complex. Kolb and Müller-Eberhard have distinguished the mechanism involved in C9 binding and activity. At low

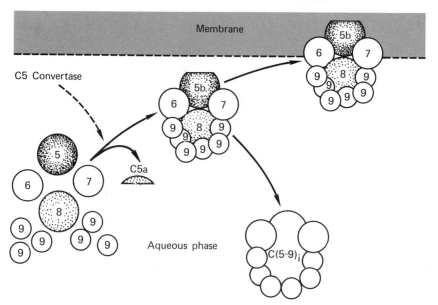

Fig. 2-2. Schematic representation of formation of a stable $(C5-9)_i$ complex. On activation of C5, association of components C5b to C9 into a firm complex ensues. This complex has the transient capacity to bind to the surface of a cell and to cause cell lysis. On loss of its binding site the stable arrangement remains in free solution without cytolytic activity. (From W. P. Kolb and H. J. Müller-Eberhard, *J. Exp. Med.,* **138**: 449, 1973.)

input levels of this component, binding is slow. The elicitation of a functional lesion, i.e., one lesion per cell or 63% lysis, requires three to six molecules of human C9. Whereas the attachment process takes place through adsorption and is insensitive to reaction temperatures, the lytic activity is highly temperature-dependent. These findings are at variance with those of Rommel and Mayer and of Kitamura and Inai who showed that only a single molecule of guinea pig or human C9 sufficed to induce a red cell lesion. Reconciliation of these conflicting reports will be awaited as an important step in clarifying the mechanism of C-mediated hemolysis.

It is important to note that this assembly of the final attack mechanism involves the nonenzymatic formation of a complex in which the components are noncovalently bound. The final enzymatic step in the classical sequence involves cleavage of C5. The larger fragment C5b is thought to initiate this assembly through a conformational change induced as a result of the limited proteolysis. A schematic representation of these mechanisms is shown in Fig. 2-3 for the membrane reactions and in Fig. 2-4 for the fluid phase events.

After the addition of C8, but not of C9, the cells exhibit a slowly evolving, low degree of lysis. This process is greatly enhanced in time and extent upon the incorporation of C9 at 37° C. Antrypol has been

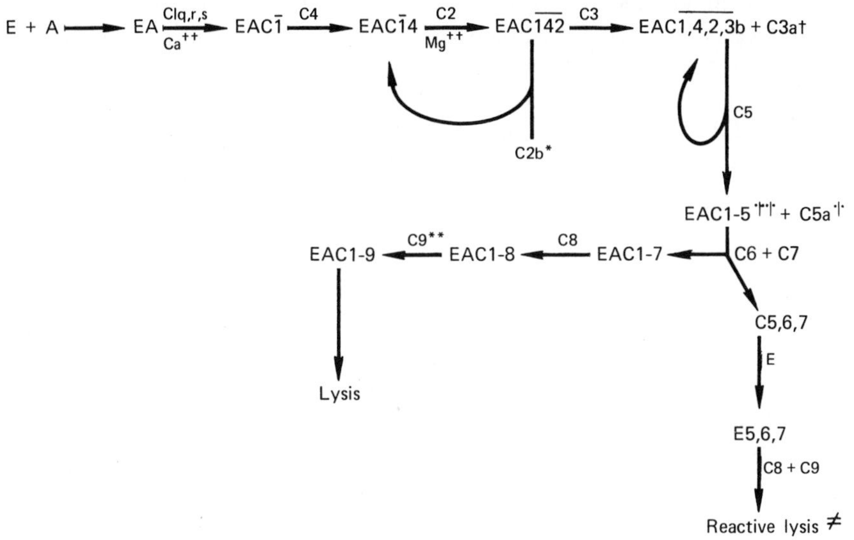

$$E + A \longrightarrow EA \xrightarrow[Ca^{++}]{C1q,r,s} EA\overline{C1} \xrightarrow{C4} EA\overline{C1}4 \xrightarrow[Mg^{++}]{C2} EA\overline{C142} \xrightarrow{C3} EA\overline{C1,4,2,3b} + C3a\dagger$$

C2b*

$$EAC1-5 \,\dagger\dagger\dagger + C5a \,\dagger$$

C5

$$EAC1-9 \xleftarrow{C9**} EAC1-8 \xleftarrow{C8} EAC1-7 \xleftarrow{} C6 + C7$$

C5,6,7

E

Lysis

E5,6,7

C8 + C9

Reactive lysis $\neq$

* Has not yet been isolated. Probably degraded by serum proteases.
† Low molecular weight peptides which do not contribute to the hemolytic sequence but possess anaphylatoxic properties.
$\neq$ Lysis of unsensitized erythrocytes by $\overline{C567}$ complex formed in fluid phase.
** Components C5 through C9 may also form a stable, hemolytically inactive C5-C9 complex in the fluid phase.
††† Ultrastructural lesions have been visualized.

Fig. 2-3. Membrane reactions. Sequence of reactions occurring on a membrane site. For E the determinant is the Forssman antigen.

(1)   C1q + C1r + C1s

$\downarrow$ Ca^{++}

$\overline{C1}$

(2) $\overline{C1}$ + C4 $\longrightarrow$ C4a* + C4b

(3) $\overline{C1}$ + C2 $\longrightarrow$ C2a + C2b*

(4) $\overline{C1}$ + $\overline{C1}$ INH $\longrightarrow$ Inactive product †

(5)   EAC42 + C3 $\longrightarrow$ C3a* + C3b

(6)   C3b + KAF (C3 INA) $\longrightarrow$ C3c* + C3d*†

(7)   EAC$\overline{4,2,3}$ + C5 $\longrightarrow$ C5a* + C5b

*Inactive fragments for the hemolytic sequence.
†May also occur with membrane-bound component.

Fig. 2-4. Some fluid phase reactions.

shown to inhibit the action of C8 and of C9. It has been postulated that C9 interacts with the C8-containing intermediate through a metal-binding site since a number of chelating agents like 1,10-phenanthroline and 2,2'-bipyridine mimic the action of C9 in terms of temperature dependence, time, and rate of the response. EDTA at relatively high concentrations (0.09 M) also inhibits the action of C9.

MECHANISM OF CYTOLYSIS

The terminal lytic process, which was originally described by Green and Goldberg in experiments with Krebs ascites tumor cells, begins with an enhanced efflux of intracellular potassium and other small molecules so that the membranes can no longer regulate the selective exchange of ions. Osmotic equilibrium is disturbed, there is an influx of water, and the cells lyse with release of their intracellular contents. When swelling of the cells is blocked, as by admixture with a relatively high concentration of serum albumin, leakage of macroglobulins may be prevented. The lesions produced in erythrocytes have been visualized by electron microscopy and negative staining as dark "holes" surrounded by lighter halos. The holes are about 10 nm in diameter when produced by human C and about 8.5 nm by guinea pig C. Each lesion has been correlated with a single site of IgM hemolysin or two IgG sites in close proximity, although evidence has been presented that several holes may be formed in the region of a single IgM site, probably due to the clustering effects of C42 and reactive lysis. The multiplicity of lesions at a single antibody site led to concern as to the validity of the one-hit theory. However, the finding that a single molecule of C9 sufficed to create a lesion and the discoveries of the clustering effect and of reactive lysis soon dispelled these doubts.

The lysis of nucleated cells seems to proceed in a manner basically similar to that of the sensitized erythrocyte. With different target cells, the degree of lysis may be influenced by the distribution of antigenic determinants on the cell membrane, the immunoglobulin class of the antibody, and the serum used as a source of complement. Interestingly, rabbit and mouse sera are more active than guinea pig serum as complement sources with nucleated cells, and these sera are more readily activated by 7S than by 19S immunoglobulins.

Mayer has recently proposed a hypothesis for the cytolytic mechanism of C, based on the lipid mosaic model of cell membranes as described by Singer. In this model, shown in Fig. 2-5, amphipathic proteins are distributed irregularly in the cell membrane, embedded in the fluid lipid bilayer. Mayer proposed that the late-acting C proteins, C5–C9, provide

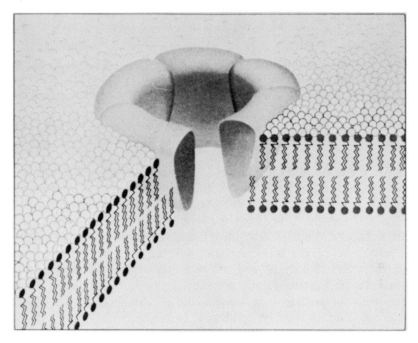

Fig. 2-5. Structure of complement lesion is depicted in schematic form. The structure is believed to consist of the five late-acting complement components C5b, C6, C7, C8 and C9. These components are thought to attach themselves to the lipid bilayer of the cell membrane. The bilayer consists of lipid molecules stacked side by side with their polar heads pointing outward and their nonpolar fatty-acid tails pointing inward. The complement components, which are proteins, are believed to assemble themselves into a doughnut or a funnel shape that penetrates the bilayer. The hollow core of the structure could form the lesion through which water and ions flow into cell until it bursts. (From M. M. Mayer, *Scientific American*, **229**: 60, 1973.)

a rigid structure at the C-activated site through which a hydrophilic channel is produced, at the termination of the C sequence, for the exchange of salts and water. This model is consistent with the following facts. If experimental conditions are selected to avoid clustering, a favorable correspondence is observed between the number of predicted holes based on titrations of the components in molecular terms and the number of lesions visualized in the electron microscope. The mass of the assembled C5–C9 complex (10^6 daltons) seems adequate for the formation of this superstructure with a channel of 100 Å in diameter. Moreover, treatment of the red cell ghosts with lipid solvents, but not with proteolytic enzymes, abolishes the holes. This feature can be rationalized with this "doughnut" model if it is assumed that the channel penetrates the entire lipid bilayer so that removal of the protruding protein structure leaves the hole relatively intact. Finally, the dark central region of the hole may represent the channel, while the surrounding lighter-staining area represents the hydrophobic portion of the amphipathic protein cylinder.

The role of lipids, though seemingly of secondary importance in this model, has been studied intensively by Kinsky with artificial membranes containing phospholipid membranes, trapped ^{14}C-glucose and the Forssman antigen, whose structure has been defined by Siddiqui and Hakomori as:

gal NAc(α1 → 3) gal NAc(β1 → 3) gal (α1 → 4) gal (β1 → 4) glc-1-ceramide

This molecule is composed of a pentasaccharide which provides the polar groups and a nonpolar region formed by sphingosine in amide linkage with a fatty acid (ceramide). The immunological specificity of this molecule is thought to reside in the terminal gal NAc residues in glycosidic linkage. Liposomes containing trapped glucose were generated by the admixture of Forssman antigen with the phospholipids lecithin or sphingomyelin, cholesterol and stearylamine or dicetyl phosphate. On treatment with Forssman antibody and C, glucose was released. Experiments with the purified nine components of human C showed that the release of glucose resembled immune hemolysis with respect to every parameter that was studied.

The data accumulated by Kinsky are entirely consistent with Singer's conception of membrane structure in the sense that the lipids provide a matrix for the assembly of the cannulated complex of C components. Kinsky showed that the release of glucose from the liposomes does not involve turnover or release of membrane phospholipids, thereby dismissing the various theories which postulated the action of phospholipases or lysolecithin in C cytolysis. The question now to be addressed concerns the mechanism of construction of the complex of C proteins in such a manner as to provide a hydrophobic exterior and an interior hydrophilic channel. The liposomes would seem to provide an excellent reagent for this type of study since they contain no adventitious proteins. The disposition of the terminal components in the postulated cylindrical superstructure may now be amenable to study in the electron microscope with ferritin-labeled antisera to the individual C components.

These considerations of cytolysis forcefully emphasize a basic aspect of C functions. For the red cell, a rather simple antigenic determinant in combination with antibody produces little change except for agglutination. The cells remain intact and functional, although they may be phagocyted more readily in the agglutinated state. Activation of the C system, however, sets into motion the complex series of events described in this chapter whose final result is cell death. It is therefore not surprising that the occurrence of these events *in vivo,* involving a variety of cells and tissues, may be associated with numerous pathological consequences.

C Inhibitors—Regulators of C Action

Like many other physiologic processes, progression of the activated C sequence is modulated by a number of homeostatic mechanisms. Some of these have already been mentioned. Thus the $\overline{C42}$ convertase of C3 and the $\overline{C4,2,3}$, or C5 convertase decay rapidly. The addition of C1 to an immune complex may be quite dissociable under physiologic conditions of temperature and ionic strength. Plasma enzymes like trypsin and plasmin may destroy components of the C system. In addition, $\overline{C1}$, $\overline{C42}$, $\overline{C423}$ cleave C4, C2, C3, and C5 respectively in the fluid phase. The self-regulating C system includes several other proteins which inactivate selected components through combination or enzymatic action.

1. $\overline{C1}$ Inhibitor ($\overline{C1}$ INH)

This is a relatively heat- and acid-labile glycoprotein of 140,000 daltons first described by Lepow and purified by Pensky from human serum. $\overline{C1}$ INH inhibits the activity of $\overline{C1s}$, but not C1 in the fluid phase or in its cell-bound state as $EAC\overline{1}$ or $EAC\overline{14}$. $\overline{C1}$ INH is thought to act by binding stoichiometrically with the $\overline{C1}$ enzyme, $C1\overline{s}$, at or near its catalytic site. Kagen and Becker noted that $\overline{C1}$ INH also inhibits the esterolytic action of plasma kallikrein, thereby establishing a link between the C system and inflammation since activation of the kallikrein system leads to bradykinin formation. Plasmin is also inhibited by $\overline{C1}$ INH providing a tie-in with blood coagulation. An inhibitor of $\overline{C1}$ has also been found in the sera of rabbits, guinea pigs, and mice.

2. C3 Inactivator (C3 INA)

Tamura and Nelson isolated a constituent from rabbit and guinea pig serum which inhibited the activity of C3b when bound to its precursor $EAC\overline{42}$. Shortly thereafter, Lachmann and Müller-Eberhard isolated a human serum constituent which also acted on cell-bound C3b so as to render the cell reactive to conglutinin. This protein, named "KAF" or conglutinogen activating factor, had properties similar to the Tamura and Nelson product. The identity of the various preparations was established by Ruddy and Austen who characterized C3 INA as a thermostable, trypsin sensitive $\beta 1$ protein with a molecular weight of 100,000 daltons. This protein resists a variety of destructive treatments. It has the ability to inactivate cell-bound C3b and therefore plays a central homeostatic role in both the classical and alternate pathways. The mode of inactivation involves proteolysis of cell-bound C3b with the presence in the fluid phase of a major fragment of C3b called C3c. The cleavage product called C3d remains on the cell-bound intermediate, thereby blocking further participation of the site in the ongoing sequence. The fragment C3c may be obtained by incubating serum at 37° C or by treatment with trypsin. C3 INA is also present in mouse serum. Antrypol (Suramin) blocks the binding site in C3b for KAF.

3. C6 *Inactivator* (C6 INA)

This inhibitor was identified by Nelson and Biro while studying the sera of rabbits which were deficient in C6. These sera and those obtained from rabbits, humans, and guinea pigs contain a protein which interfered with the functioning of cell-bound C6. C6 INA is a discrete molecule separable from C6 by ultracentrifugation and chromatography. Like the C3 INA, the C6 inhibitor acts only on the cell-bound component by preventing the addition of C7. Neither inhibitor affects fluid-phase components or intermediates.

CONGLUTININ AND IMMUNOCONGLUTININ

The phenomenon of conglutination—the intense agglutination of erythrocytes by bovine serum following their interaction with antibody and complement—came under serious study during the first decade of this century. The term conglutinin (K) is given to a nonimmunoglobulin protein found in normal sera of mammals. The conglutinating activity found in cattle serum is due to the reaction of this protein with conglutinogen, a heat-stable mannan-peptide found in yeast cell walls, zymosan, and on cell surfaces containing bound complement of many species. Equine serum is particularly rich in conglutinogen. When purified preparations of conglutinin and conglutinogen are added to fresh serum, fixation of C1 and of hemolytic is demonstrable. This reaction is best demonstrated with rabbit serum as the C source. Human serum is less effective and guinea pig serum is but weakly reactive.

The term immunoconglutinin designates an antibody formed to C components fixed *in vivo* on immune complexes. It therefore represents an immune response by the host to "hidden determinants" of autologous C components that have become cell-bound *in vivo*. They are generally of the IgM class and are detected by agglutination of erythrocytes carrying various intermediates of the C sequence. Thus, immunoconglutinin formed in humans will agglutinate EAC4 and, particularly, EAC43 and EAC43b. Immunoconglutinin activity has also been found in human saliva. As Lachmann has stated, ". . . there is little doubt that immunoconglutinin formation to a large extent mirrors *in vivo* C fixation (but) the evidence that immunoconglutinins serve a significant adaptive function is not compelling." Data are available, however, to suggest that immunoconglutinin enhances C activities associated with host defense mechanisms such as phagocytosis and the bactericidal activity of serum.

FURTHER READING

Ingram, D. C. (ed.), *Biological Activities of Complement*, S. Karger, Basel, 1972.

Kabat, E. A., and Mayer, M. M., *Experimental Immunochemistry*, C. C. Thomas & Co., Springfield, Ill., 1961. Chapter 4 deals with Complement and Complement Fixation.

Kolb, W. P., and Müller-Eberhard, H. J., "The Membrane Attack Mechanism of Complement," *J. Exp. Med.* **141**:724, 1975.

Lachmann, P. J., "Conglutinin and Immunoconglutinins," *Adv. Immunology,* **6**:479, 1967.

Lepow, I. H., Dias da Silva, W., and Patrick, R. A., "Biologically Active Cleavage Products of Components of Complement," in *Cellular and Humoral Mechanisms in Anaphylaxis and Allergy,* H. Z. Movat (ed.), S. Karger, Basel, 1969, p. 237.

Mayer, M. M., "Mechanism of Cytolysis by Complement," *Proc. Nat'l Acad. Sci. U.S.A.,* **69**:2954, 1972.

Mayer, M. M., Osler, A. G., Bier, O. G., and Heidelberger, M., "The Activating Effect of Magnesium and Other Cations on the Hemolytic Function of Complement," *J. Exp. Med.,* **84**:535, 1946.

Müller-Eberhard, H. J., in The Harvey Lectures, Series 66, pp. 75–104, 1970–71.

Müller-Eberhard, H. J., "Complement," *Ann. Rev. Biochem.,* **38**:389, 1969.

Nelson, R. A., Jr., Jensen, J., Gigli, I., and Tamura, N., "Methods for the Separation, Purification and Measurement of Nine Components of the Hemolytic Complement in Guinea Pig Serum," *Immunochemistry,* **3**:111, 1966.

"Nomenclature of Complement," *Immunochemistry,* **7**:137–142, 1970.

Rapp, H. J., and Borsos, T., *Molecular Basis of Complement Action,* Appleton-Century-Crofts, New York, 1970.

Schreiber, R. D., and Müller-Eberhard, H. J., "Fourth Component of Human Complement: Description of a Three Polypeptide Chain Structure," *J. Exp. Med.,* **140**:1324, 1974.

Schultz, D. R., *The Complement System,* S. Karger, Basel, 1971.

Shelton, E., Yonemasi, K., and Stroud, R. M., "Ultrastructure of the Human Complement Component, $C1_q$," *Proc. Nat'l Acad. Sci. U.S.A.,* **69**:65, 1972.

Chapter 3

Alternate Complement Pathways

An important advance in C research during the past few years has been the rediscovery and widespread acceptance of the fact that the C system can be activated by a variety of stimuli through alternate pathways which initiate a sequence that does not require participation of the early-acting components, C1, C4, and C2. Historically, this concept arose from experiments reported during the first two decades of this century which showed that the hemolytic action of C was destroyed by treatment of fresh serum with cobra venom or yeast. The finding that this inactivation involved the component then called C′3 laid the basis for the use of the so-called R reagents to define the mechanism of C action. These reagents consisted of serum subjected to various treatments such that they were then thought to lack only a single component while supplying an excess of the remainder. Thus, at the time when only four components were recognized, the reagent R3 was used to supply C′1, C′4, and C′2 without contributing C′3 activity. R1, R2, and R4 reagents were prepared in analogous fashion. These preparations were used by Pillemer, Lepow, and their associates in studies which suggested that the destruction of C′3 by zymosan (a suspension of boiled yeast cell walls) was not simply an adsorption process as previously thought. A complex enzymatic process was envisioned due to the temperature, Mg^{++}, ionic strength and pH requirements for restitution of immune hemolysis. Further work by this group led to the identification of a serum protein called Properdin (P), and the hypothesis was formulated that normal serum contained a second lytic system comprising properdin, Factor A (sensitive to primary amines), Factor B (heat-labile), and magnesium. Great interest was aroused by these reports since the scope of action of this system excluded the participation of antibody despite its capacity to kill gram-negative bacteria, neutralize viruses, lyse erythrocytes obtained from patients with paroxysmal nocturnal hemoglobinuria (PNH), and protect animals against ionizing radiation. In view of the broad range of activity and lack of specificity ascribed to the properdin system, experimental and theoretical challenges were soon forthcoming.

The essential steps in the reaction between serum and zymosan were thought to be:

1. $Z + P$ (in fresh normal serum) $\xrightarrow[17°C]{Mg^{++}}$ PZ

2. PZ + fresh serum (Factors A and B) + Mg^{++} $\xrightarrow{37°C}$ Inactivation of C′3 in which P refers to properdin, Z to zymosan, and PZ to the properdin-zymosan complex which, in the presence of serum factors A and B, selectively inactivated C′3.

Several assumptions, inherent in the proposed mechanism of properdin action, were quick to attract critical appraisal. The thesis that the broad spectrum of properdin activities did not involve specific antibody and the early C components was challenged by Nelson. He observed that the preferential reactivity of zymosan with C′3 could be duplicated in reaction systems with low levels of antibody to bovine serum albumin or pneumococci. Moreover, the zymosan reaction with serum also diminished the activities of C1 and C4. In addition, several investigators demonstrated that the bactericidal action attributed to the nonspecific properties of the properdin system was associated with the presence of specific antibodies. In retrospect, it was inevitable that these and other interpretational uncertainties delayed the ready acceptance of the properdin theory as initially proposed. These problems were created by the nature of the assay systems and the use of immunologically impure reagents. For example, the reagent then called C′3 is now known to have comprised at least six different activities, since it contained C3, C5, C6, C7, C8, and C9. Rigorous standardization of the RP reagents could not therefore be achieved, particularly in titrations whose endpoint fluctuated over a twofold range. The role of magnesium could not be adequately explained without implicating C2, since this cofactor was shown to be essential for the participation of this component in immune hemolysis. Attempts to establish the null hypothesis that normal serum lacks immunoglobulins to antigenic determinants on bacterial or yeast cell walls have since been discarded, particularly as a result of the extensive cross reactions in plant and animal cells demonstrated by Heidelberger and by Springer. Nor was the possibility entertained by those who discovered the properdin system or by those who denied its existence that the inactivation of C′3, the lysis of red cells, and the destruction of gram-negative bacteria could indeed be mediated by two different mechanisms, only one of which required specific antibody.

Fortunately, this controversy has now been resolved with the aid of the purified complement components and the discovery in several laboratories of alternate pathways of C activation. As a result, the views of Pillemer, Lepow, and their colleagues, maintained over a period spanning two decades, have now been thoroughly vindicated and several of the major components of this reaction sequence have been characterized.

CONSTITUENTS OF THE PROPERDIN SYSTEM

A homogeneous protein with the properties ascribed earlier to properdin has been isolated from human serum by Pensky, Lepow, and their co-workers and subsequently in other laboratories. It is described as a 5.2S γ2 basic glycoprotein of 185,000 daltons with a carbohydrate content of 9.8%. When isolated by affinity chromatography or by elution from complexes formed with zymosan, the properdin preparations seem to contain four noncovalently bound units, each of 46,000 daltons. These preparations were homogeneous as judged by molecular sieve filtration, ultracentrifugation, and electrophoresis on alkaline polyacrylamide gels and immunological procedures. They had a high content of glycine and proline, thus resembling C1q. Purified properdin had no activity attributable to the classical C components nor did it agglutinate zymosan particles, suggesting a lack of antibody activity. Moreover, rabbit antisera to human IgG, IgM, IgA, or light chains failed to react with properdin. On the positive side, the purified preparations of properdin, in the presence of the other cofactors, mediated some of the reactions previously ascribed to the system, i.e., lysis of erythrocytes from patients with paroxysmal nocturnal hemoglobinuria and killing of *Shigella dysenteriae*. Specific antiserum to properdin has been produced and used in a radioimmunoassay which will undoubtedly be useful in studies of the role of this reagent in various types of tissue damage. The fact that as little as 10 μg of properdin suffice to inactivate about 50% of the hemolytic activity of C3 in a milliliter of fresh serum emphasizes the potential biological importance of the properdin system.

The difficulties previously associated with properdin assays based on its action in the hemolytic system have been surmounted by the radioimmunoassay designed by Minta, Goodkofsky, and Lepow. This assay is based on the principle of competitive binding between properdin in the test sample and radioiodinated purified properdin for the specific antibody. As shown in Fig. 3-1, estimates of serum properdin levels are obtained by

Fig. 3-1. Inhibition of binding of 40 ng ^{125}I properdin to antiproperdin coated tubes by (a) increasing concentrations of unlabeled properdin, (b) increasing dilutions of normal human serum. Polystyrene tubes were coated at 23°C for 2 hr with 1 ml rabbit anti-human properdin diluted 1:1000. The antibody coated tubes were equilibrated at 37°C for 5 (●——●), 9 (○——○) and 24 hr (▲——▲) with 10–100 ng of unlabeled properdin or serum dilutions (1/300–1/1400) in 0.5% BSA. The contents of the tubes were aspirated and replaced with 40 ng ^{125}I properdin in 0.5% BSA and reincubated at 37°C for a further period of 24 hr. The tubes were counted, rinsed, and recounted to determine the bound radioactivity. (From J. O. Minta et al., *Immunochemistry*, **10**: 341, 1973.) BSA = Bovine serum albumin.

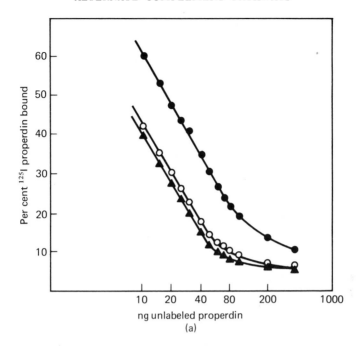

ng unlabeled properdin

(a)

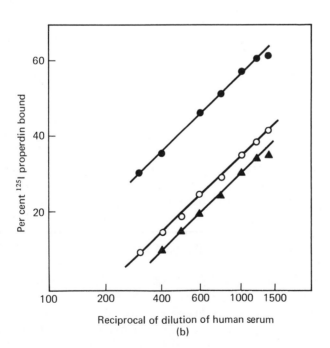

Reciprocal of dilution of human serum

(b)

interpolation on a standard reference curve constructed with varying amounts of the purified preparation. Sera of normal individuals contain 17.2–29.4 μg of properdin/ml with a mean value of 24.7 ± 3.9 μg/ml.

The properdin assay was developed shortly after a number of reports from several laboratories described alternate pathways of C activation which had features in common with the original properdin system. Since these findings all came to light at about the same time, they will be summarized in terms of reaction mechanisms now generally accepted but still under active investigation. One of the central components in this scheme, originally called GBG and C3PA, now known to be Factor B, was isolated in several laboratories.

This properdin system reactant was identified in the early studies as a heat-labile substance, destroyed at 50° C for 30 minutes, which cooperated with properdin and Factor A in the inactivation of C3. Several independent approaches have led to its further characterization. Haupt and Heide, and later Boenisch and Alper, had isolated a β-glycoprotein from normal human serum called β_2-glycoprotein and glycine-rich β-glycoprotein, respectively. Although the identities of these two proteins were soon established, their biological properties were not fully appreciated until somewhat later.

The importance of this protein in host defense processes became apparent in studies of a patient with heightened susceptibility to bacterial infections by Alper, Rosen, Abramson, and their associates. Laboratory studies indicated that important C functions such as the mediation of bactericidal and phagocytic reactions were absent despite the fact that the hemolytic activity of the patient's serum was only moderately reduced (15 CH_{50} per ml as compared to the normal range of 40 ± 5 CH_{50} per ml). The reduction in hemolytic activity was associated with decreased C3 activity. All the remaining components were at normal levels as judged by hemolytic and immunochemical studies. C3 levels were assayed immunochemically at 280 μg/ml, about one-fourth the normal value, but only about a quarter of this quantity possessed the electrophoretic mobility of native C3. The mobility of the remainder was characteristic of the C3b split product. Of singular significance was the observation that the addition of C3 to the patient's serum failed to restore the missing C functions. Since the newly supplied C3 was quickly converted *in vivo* to its inactive C3b form, a search was initiated for a C3-cleaving enzyme. This was soon found and called GBGase, since it cleaved the glycine-rich β-glycoprotein or GBG. Additional abnormalities were found in this patient's serum, namely, a complete lack of GBG due to the absence of a GBGase inhibitor. This enzyme was isolated from normal serum as a 6S heat-labile pseudoglobulin. The fact that the activity of GBGase was Mg^{++}-dependent and that GBG was unstable at 37° C suggested an alternate C pathway reminiscent of the properdin system. The relationship of GBG to properdin was quickly established by the collaborative efforts of Alper, Goodkofsky, and Lepow, through which it became apparent that GBG was in fact properdin Factor B. This conclusion was based on similarities in dose-response curves, electrophoretic properties, and in their biological functions as inactivators of C components.

The converging lines of evidence which equated GBG with properdin Factor B had still another dimension. In the mid-sixties a number of investigators independently extended earlier findings regarding the destruction of C3 in serum treated with cobra venom. The active component in the venom was found to be a glycoprotein (140,000 daltons) which inactivated C3 in serum but not in reaction mixtures containing only purified C3 and the cobra venom glycoprotein. This observation stimulated the search for the other serum factors and uncovered a thermolabile, 5S pseudoglobulin with β-mobility and a molecular weight of 80,000. This protein, called C3PA for C3 proactivator, was shown to combine with the cobra venom factor (CoF) in the presence of still other serum factors to form a complex that fragmented C3. It was therefore a C3 convertase whose natural substrate was the same as the $\overline{C42}$ convertase, but which differed in its constituents and mode of assembly. The presentations and discussions at the 5th International Complement Workshop in 1973 and comparative experiments by several investigators removed all doubts that the C3PA isolated in Müller-Eberhard's laboratory had the functional and immunochemical properties of GBG and properdin Factor B. On this basis, it would be historically appropriate to retain the name Factor B for this component of the alternate pathway.

The mounting evidence for the existence of the properdin system was further strengthened by the demonstration that one of its reactants, the hydrazine-sensitive Factor A was in fact C3. It had been known for many years that the activity of C3 as well as that of C4 was abrogated by treatment with hydrazine and other primary amines. However, the decision that Factor A was one or the other of these C components awaited the availability of purified component preparations. Two types of experiments established the identity of Factor A as C3. In one, the presence of hydrazine in reaction mixtures containing Factor B (C3PA) and inulin-activated serum (see below) prevented the cleavage of C3. This inhibition was overcome with an additional input of C3. Secondly, dose-response curves describing the hemolytic action of C3 and the function of Factor A were quantitatively superimposable in terms of their inhibition by hydrazine. Graded amounts of this amine destroyed both activities to the same extent. Moreover, quantitative restoration of both activities was achieved with C3 but not with C4.

This brief resume of the history of the properdin system and its current resurrection is of interest from several viewpoints and firmly establishes the individuality of this C activation system. The story is not yet complete since additional factors have been implicated and some of their mechanistic aspects are still under study.

In the course of their studies of the patient with congenital hyper-catabolism of C3, Boenisch and Alper concluded that serum contained an enzymatic activity (GBGase) capable of cleaving GBG (Factor B or C3PA) and that their patient's serum lacked an inhibitor of this proteolytic reaction. Müller-Eberhard and Götze, and later Austen and his colleagues, isolated this enzyme, now called Factor D, C3PAse, or Factor B convertase. They characterized this protein as a 3S α-globulin of 25,000 daltons, which differed from the 4S α-globulin, $C\overline{1s}$, in terms of its enzymatic and antigenic properties.

As indicated, the terms Factor B and Factor D are synonymous with C3PA and C3PAse, respectively. Of considerable importance in this scheme is the demonstration that conversion of the precursor C3PA to its active form, C3 Activator or $\overline{B}$, requires metal ions and a C3 fragment which has been identified as C3b. The C3b fragment thus appears to provide the means for a positive feedback mechanism. Factor D is present in serum as an inert enzyme precursor which may be activated by treatment with tryp-sin. Under physiologic conditions, conversion of the precursor to its enzy-matic form occurs through its interaction with C3b, a step modulated by P. The D enzyme ($\overline{D}$) or C3PAse is inhibitable by diisopropylfluorophosphate and by the synthetic amino acid ester, p-tosyl-l-arginine methyl ester (TAMe). It is therefore classified as a serine esterase.

The conversion of Factor B to an enzyme which splits C3 seems then to be multi-unit in structure containing P, D, and C3b as illustrated in Fig. 3-2.

Most recently another properdin system factor has been isolated from the plasma of patients with hypocomplementemic chronic glomerulonephri-tis. The activation of this factor called C3NeF, is thought to constitute the initial step in the assembly of the complex enzyme which splits C3.

The homeostatic mechanism for the cycle of C3b participation in the conversion of Factor B to the C3 convertase, $\overline{B}$ or C3 Activator, also involves the reagent called KAF, the conglutinogen-activating factor dis-cussed in the previous chapter. This plasma constituent converts conglu-tinogen into conglutinin, a molecular entity which agglutinates erythrocytes containing fixed C3, C3b. KAF induces proteolysis of C3b into the cell-bound fragment C3d and an antigenically distinct fragment C3c which is shed from the cells. Fragmentation of C3b may also occur in the fluid phase. KAF, sometimes called C3b inactivator, first described by Tamura and Nelson, has also been studied by Lachmann and his colleagues and by Ruddy and Austen. The role of this inhibitor, apparently lacking in the serum of Alper and Rosen's patient with congenital hypercatabolism of C3, has been recently clarified by Nicol and Lachmann. These investigators

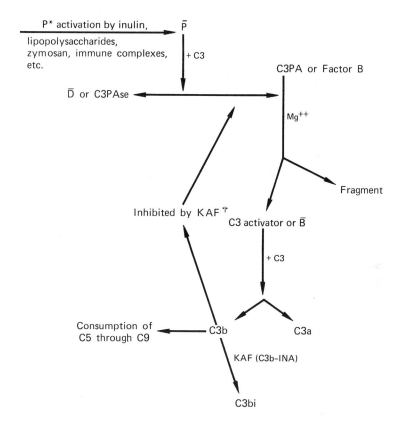

*Recent evidence suggests that the conversion of P to $\bar{P}$ is preceded by the activation of another serum proenzyme, the C3 nephritic factor (C3Ne$\underline{F}$) which then acts on P. It is also thought that activation of D to $\bar{D}$ requires the participation of properdin.
† Now termed C3b-INA

Fig. 3-2. Postulated sequence of the properdin pathway, also called the alternate or alternative pathway.

found that the *in vitro* action of KAF accurately mimics the *in vivo* effects by converting C3b to its inactive form and by inhibiting the proteolysis of C3PA, thereby effectively terminating the sequence leading to the formation of C3 Activator, $\bar{B}$. In side reactions which may overcome inhibition by KAF, it should be mentioned that C3b can also be generated from C3 by a variety of non-C-dependent enzymes which include thrombin, plasmin, and other sera, tissue and lysosomal proteases. The studies with KAF provided firm evidence regarding the positive feedback role assigned to C3b. The properties of the properdin system components are listed in Table 3-1 and their postulated mode of action is depicted in Fig. 3-2.

Table 3–1

Components of the alternate (properdin) reaction sequence

Component	Synonyms	Concentration in serum, $\mu g/ml$	Molecular weight	Function
Properdin		25	185,000	Participates with C3 (Factor A), C3PAse (C3PA convertase), and Factor B (C3PA) in cleaving C3 into C3a and C3b.
C3	Hydrazine sensitive factor; Factor A	1230	195,000	Substrate for $\overline{C42}$ of the classical system and $\overline{B}$ of the alternate pathway.
C3PAse	GBGAse; Factor D	trace	24,000	A 3S α-globulin which is Mg^{++}-dependent and with activated properdin converts C3PA to C3A ($\overline{B}$) with loss of a minor fragment.
C3PA	C3 proactivator; Factor B; GBG; β_2 glycoprotein 2	100–200	93,000	Precursor of C3A ($\overline{B}$), a C3 convertase.
C3A	C3 activator, $\overline{B}$		63,000	The enzyme which splits C3 into C3b and C3a.
C3b				Major fragment of cleaved C3 serving a positive feedback role in the conversion of C3PA to C3A.
KAF	Conglutinogen activating factor; C3b inactivator, C3b-INA			Cleaves C3b to C3bi, rendering C3b inactive with release of C3c.

ACTIVATION OF THE PROPERDIN SYSTEM

The discussion of the properdin system has thus far failed to consider the initial steps which trigger this complex sequence. Although some information has been gained as to the nature of the triggering agents, the mechanism of the early steps is still unclear. Indeed, we still lack adequate data as to the precise step in the sequence at which properdin participates in the events leading to the formation of C3 Activator, B. In the discussion which follows as to the nature of the triggering agents, the possibility is not excluded that there may be several reaction steps, one of which involves C3NeF, which precede the conversion of properdin into its activated form.

As indicated, most of the early experiments by the Pillemer group were based on the interaction of fresh serum with yeast cell wall particles, i.e., zymosan. Interpretational confusion arose from the inability to clearly distinguish between an antibody-mediated event and another mode of activation involving properdin, both of which lead to C3 destruction. Similar considerations were applicable to the experiments in which cell walls from gram-negative or gram-positive bacteria and high molecular weight polysaccharides were substituted for zymosan under *in vitro* or *in vivo* conditions. It is reasonable to conclude at this writing that both mechanisms, i.e., antibody and properdin, are stimulated by the admixture of microbial cell walls with fresh serum. The experiments of Gewurz and his collaborators are instructive in this regard as shown in Fig. 3-3. These data indicate that the addition of an immune aggregate (bovine serum albumin and its antibody) to fresh serum leads to activity reductions in each of the nine complement components, with substantial fixation of C1, C4, and C2. This profile differs materially from that obtained upon the addition of zymosan or the endotoxic lipopolysaccharide from the gram-negative bacterium, *Veillonella alcalescens*. In the latter two instances, there is abundant consumption of the overall hemolytic activity of the serum with but minimal losses of C1, C4, or C2 activity. Inactivation of the six terminal components (C3–C9) proceeds in a manner generally similar to that observed with the immune aggregates.

The profiles depicted in Fig. 3-3 clearly suggest that at least two modes of C destruction are induced in the lipopolysaccharide (LPS)-serum interaction. The slight losses of C1, C4, and C2 obtained with the cell walls of bacteria or yeast probably reflect mediation by low levels of specific or cross-reacting antibodies in the sera. Evidence for this interpretation has recently been provided by Fine and by Loos and collaborators. In the former instance, red cells coated with LPS were lysed in the presence of normal serum. The incorporation of ethyleneglycol tetraacetate (EGTA) inhibited destruction of the LPS-coated cells. It is well established that

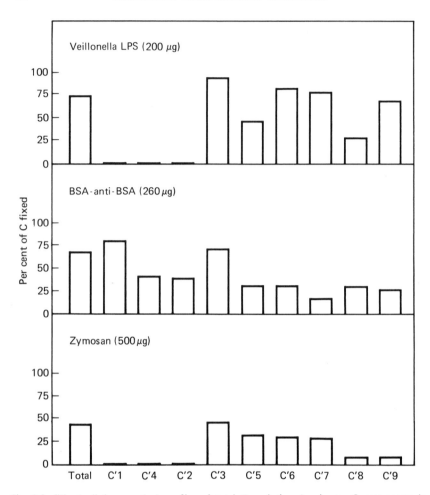

Fig. 3-3. "Fixation" (consumption) profiles of total C and the nine known C components in concentrated guinea pig serum (0.9 ml in a total volume of 1.0 ml) upon interaction with 200 μg *Veillonella alcalescens* lipopolysaccharide (LPS), 260 μg washed preformed immune complexes of bovine serum albumin (BSA) and rabbit antiserum (anti-BSA) reacted at equivalence, and 500 μg zymosan during 1 hr incubation at 37°C. Current usage dispenses with the superscripts. Thus C'1, C'4, etc., are now called C1, C4 respectively. (From H. Gewurz, H. S. Shin, and S. Mergenhagen, *J. Exp. Med.*, 128: 1052, 1968.)

this chelating agent suppresses the classical C system by binding calcium. EGTA does not interfere with alternate pathway activity since sufficient magnesium is still available. Moreover, the experiments of Loos and others showed that LPS preparations from different organisms varied in their capacity to inhibit purified $\overline{C1}$. No inhibition was obtained with an LPS prepared from a rough salmonella organism. With preparations from smooth forms, the extent of inhibition ranged from 16 to 98%. The suppression of $C\bar{1}$ activity is attributed to the formation of insoluble aggregates formed by LPS, antibody, and C1q.

The activity profile resulting from activation of the properdin system differs from the antibody-dependent mechanism in several important features in addition to the differences shown in Fig. 3-3. Thus induction of C activation by lipopolysaccharides is markedly temperature-dependent and, unlike the requirements of immune complexes, does not progress well with diluted serum. The participation of properdin is also consistent with the observation that endotoxins are active with sera obtained from man or other animals with immunodeficiency states. As Gewurz points out, the newborn precolostral piglet circulates less than 2.5×10^{-6} gm of gamma globulin, yet this serum supports C activation by lipopolysaccharides. However sera from these animals or hypogammaglobulinemic humans generally possess diminished C activity. The endotoxic lipopolysaccharides are also less efficient in these sera, so it is not possible to exclude a role for antibody in these experiments.

The participation of properdin in reaction mixtures containing zymosan or bacterial lipopolysaccharides and fresh serum was definitely established by Müller-Eberhard and co-workers who demonstrated cleavage of Factor B under these conditions. The sera of guinea pigs with an absolute deficiency of C4 also support C consumption by LPS, albeit to a lesser extent. Finally, experiments in Mayer's laboratory showed that the Fab fragments of a potent antiserum to C2 suppressed the activity of the $C\overline{42}$ C3 convertase but did not impede the cleavage of C3 by lipopolysaccharides. These investigators confirmed Gewurz's finding that small amounts of C2 are utilized in the interaction of endotoxin with fresh serum. They have extended these findings with efforts to isolate and characterize the enzymatic activities present on zymosan particles after treatment with guinea pig sera. They found that following this treatment zymosan probably combines with several serum components and that these complexes can cleave purified C3 as well as C5. The complexes evidently contain two multi-unit enzymatic activities in view of the kinetic differences in substrate utilization (C3 as compared to C5) and their different rates of decay at 37° C. Both complexes contain Factor B. It is very likely that these complexes contain both the $C\overline{42}$ and $C\overline{4,2,3}$ convertases of the classical system formed with antibody to zymosan as well as the C3 and C5 splitting enzymes of the alternate pathway involving properdin. These enzymes are formed much more rapidly in normal guinea pig serum than in C4-deficient serum, again suggesting utilization of both complement activation pathways in accord with interpretation of the data in Fig. 3-3. An important finding in these experiments was the presence of C3b as one of the constituents in the C3- and C5-cleaving enzymes.

Since zymosan-bound C3b accelerated the assembly of these multi-unit enzymes and fluid-phase C3b did not, it was suggested that C3b may have dual functions in the properdin system, i.e., fuel a feedback mechanism and provide one constituent for the multi-unit enzyme assembled on zymosan.

A current application of the early reports by Pillemer's group is found in the use of inulin as an activator of the alternate pathway. Suspensions of this polyfructose have been used as a simple and convenient reagent for setting the properdin sequence into motion and delineating the reaction sequence. Under the experimental conditions used by Götze and Müller-Eberhard, consumption of the terminal components (C5–C9) without a loss of C2 has been observed upon addition of inulin. It is of interest, however, that solutions rather than suspensions of this polysaccharide may be inhibitory; thus a mixed effect may be obtained in experiments based on activation of the alternate pathway by inulin.

Several of the recent advances in our understanding of the properdin system emerged from studies of its activation by antigen-antibody complexes in the author's laboratory. The experiments which demonstrated this pathway stemmed from our interest in the apparent lack of C fixation by guinea pig IgG1 immunoglobulins in contrast to the activity of the IgG2 antibodies. These differences were revealed in C fixation protocols based on the use of highly diluted guinea pig C, e.g., 1% or less. We reinvestigated these findings by first preparing large pools of each of the immunoglobulin subclasses, free of mutual contamination. C-fixation experiments were then performed with undiluted guinea pig serum as a C source. With a relatively low antibody input, e.g., 1 to 10 μg of antibody N per ml, no fixation of C was observed with the IgG1 immunoglobulins when the order of addition was antibody, C, and antigen. When this sequence was reversed by adding antibody and antigen so that ample opportunity was provided for complex formation to proceed before admixture with C, fixation was observed, particularly with the larger amounts of antibody. The IgG2 immunoglobulins were active regardless of the order of reagent addition. Further studies showed that activation of the C system by the preformed immune aggregates composed of IgG1 and specific antigen progressed with little or no consumption of the hemolytic activity of C1 or C2 but with marked utilization of C3 and the later components. The C-fixing properties of the preformed IgG1 complexes but not of the incipient aggregates recalled a similar finding made some 15 years earlier with Dr. Ovary regarding the ability of equine immunoglobulins to consume the hemolytic function of rat C and to generate anaphylatoxins. We then considered the possibility that the preformed aggregates were biologically active because a C-fixing site other than that on the Fc fragment exposed receptor sites for a serum enzyme which was not part of the classical C sequence but which utilized C3 as its natural substrate. In the search for this site, we prepared gamma-1 and gamma-2 antibodies to a DNP-protein conjugate and treated portions of these preparations with pepsin to destroy the intact Fc piece, leaving the divalent $F(ab')_2$ fragments. C-fixation reactions with preformed aggregates containing these antibodies revealed that the gamma-2 molecules had two C-activation sites, one on the Fc piece for the classical pathway and another on the $F(ab')_2$ dimer for the alternate pathway. The data plotted in Fig. 3-4 show that the native or pepsin-treated gamma-1 immunoglobulins produced identical dose-response C-fixation curves. This was not the case for the gamma-2 antibodies which yielded two distinctly different dose-response relationships, depending upon the presence of the intact preparations containing the Fc piece or the pepsin-digested Fab dimers in the immune complexes. The enzyme-treated preparations for the gamma-1 and gamma-2 immunoglobulins fixed C in precisely the same fashion with respect to their dose-response relationships and their avoidance of C1, C4, and C2 during the C-activation process, as shown in Table 3-2. These data coupled with

Table 3–2

Fixation of complement components by preformed immune aggregates in hyperimmune guinea pig antisera and HSA *

Antibody fraction †	Amount ‡	Percent activity lost									
		C	C1	C4	C2	C3	C5	C6	C7	C8	C9
	µg N										
A (IgG2)	100	>90	>99	94	65	>95	46	42	45	15	25
	25	>90	75	75	57	>95	47	45	33	11	21
	6	55	30	10	19	92	23	20	24	7	14
H (IgG1)	113	50	0	0	19	90	20	15	24	1	10
	26	47	0	0	0	83	6	21	12	1	16
	6.5	38	0	0	0	66		13	9	1	12

* From A. L. Sandberg, A. G. Osler, H. S. Shin, and B. Oliveira, J. Immunol., 104:332, 1970.
† Formed at ratios of guinea pig A (IgG2) to HSA N = 5 and guinea pig H (IgG1) N to HSA N = 5.7. The terms IgG1 and γ1, and IgG2 and γ2 are interchangeable.
‡ Anti-HSA N/ml of undiluted guinea pig serum used as complement (1.0 ml C used).

those in Fig. 3-4 clarified the results of earlier experiments in which the essential role of the Fc piece for the fixation of C had been questioned. As shown in Table 3-2, the utilization of the C components by the two antibody preparations was quite dissimilar. The gamma-2 molecules traversed the classic C pathway while their gamma-1 counterparts enter the sequence at the C3 step, without consuming the early-acting components, C1, C4, and C2. A number of other differences have been identified in

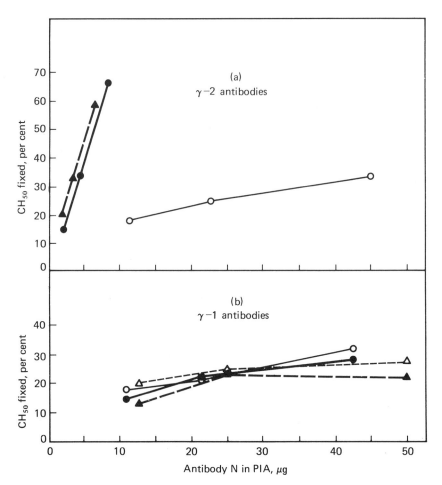

Fig. 3-4. Fixation of guinea pig complement by homologous γ-1 and γ-2 immunoglobulins. A, γ-2 antibodies: ▲ , DEAE preparation, untreated; ● , purified preparation, untreated; O , purified preparation, after pepsin digestion. B, γ-1 antibodies: ▲ , DEAE preparation, untreated; Δ , DEAE preparation, after pepsin digestion; ● , purified preparation, untreated; O , purified preparation, after pepsin digestion. All preparations were tested as preformed immune aggregates (PIA) precipitated at equivalence zone ratios of antibody to antigen. (From A. L. Sandberg, B. Oliveira, and A. G. Osler, Two Complement Interaction Sites in Guinea Pig Immunoglobulins, J. Immunol., **106**: 284, 1971.)

the parameters governing these two modes of C fixation. They are listed in Table 3-3.

The availability of multiple pathways of C activation by immune aggregates became apparent concurrently with the finding of Factor B (C3PA) activity in human sera. It was therefore of considerable interest

Table 3–3

Comparative properties of the alternate (properdin) and classical systems of complement activation *

	Alternate or properdin system	Classical system
1. Activating immunoglobulins	Human, rabbit, and guinea pig IgG, hu IgA and hu IgE	Human IgM and IgG1, IgG2 and IgG3, IgM and IgG of other species
2. Activation site	F(ab')$_2$ or Fc piece	Fc piece only
3. Participation of early-acting components	None	Essential
4. Participation of late-acting components beginning with C3	Yes	Yes
5. Functional in C4-deficient guinea pigs	Yes	No
6. Divalent cation requirements	Magnesium	Calcium and magnesium
7. Inhibited by EDTA	Yes	Yes
8. Inhibited by EGTA	No	Yes
9. C3-cleaving enzyme	The C3 proactivator-derived, C3 Activator or $\overline{B}$	The C3 convertase, $\overline{C42}$
10. Serum concentration dependence for C fixation	Lower efficiency on dilution	Greater relative efficiency on dilution
11. Temperature optimum for C fixation	37°C †	4°C
12. Time course	Generally more rapid	Usually slower
13. Inhibitable by salicylaldoxime	>50% at 0.005 M	None at 0.02 M
14. Activatable by Mg^{++}, Mn^{++} or Co^{++}	Yes	No. Ca^{++} essential

* From A. G. Osler and A. L. Sandberg, *Prog. in Allergy,* 17:51, 1973.

† A recent report indicates that the alternate pathway may be activated by IgA after incubation with serum at 0°C for 8 hours.

to ascertain whether one or more common reaction steps characterized the immune and inulin activation mechanisms. In collaboration with Drs. Götze and Müller-Eberhard, it was found that both triggering agents led to conversion of C3PA to C3 Activator with consumption of the late-acting components as shown in Table 3-4.

The significance of these results stems from the demonstration that Factor B (C3PA) can be converted to a C3-splitting enzyme under physiologic conditions in a manner seemingly consistent with the action of endotoxin and inulin. It is not yet clear whether the initial reaction steps involving properdin are identical with these three reagents, but the

Table 3—4

Conversion of C3PA and cleavage of C3 by aggregates of
gamma-1 and gamma-2 guinea pig anti-DNP.BGG *

	Conversion of C3PA, percent ‡	Cleavage of C3, percent ‡
Intact gamma-2 †	60	>80
F(ab')$_2$ of gamma-2	20	25
Intact gamma-1	40	50
F(ab')$_2$ of gamma-1	10	25

* From A. L. Sandberg, O. Götze, H. J. Müller-Eberhard, and A. G. Osler, *J. Immunol.*, 107:920, 1971.

† All aggregates contained 26 $\pm$ 1 μg of antibody N at near equivalence zone ratios.

‡ As judged by immunoelectrophoretic analyses.

elucidation of these early steps involving immune complexes are currently under study.

Before discussing other means of alternate pathway activation, it should be noted that the postulated modes of interaction of the alternate pathway sequence as shown in Table 3-1 and Fig. 3-2 represent very recent developments. It is therefore necessary to stress the possibility that these data may be incomplete in the sense that the active pace of current research may uncover additional components, new intermediates, and new reaction steps. Some, like the recent description of a properdin convertase and the experiments describing the multi-unit enzymes which split C3 and C5, have been mentioned. Thus, while it is generally accepted that the conversion of properdin to its activated state takes place early in the sequence, its mechanism and precise localization in the sequence is not yet clear.

An important point to note is that the completion of the sequence shown in Fig. 3-2 does not result in the lysis of unsensitized erythrocytes except with those from patients with paroxysmal noctural hemoglobinuria (PNH). The basis for the increased susceptibility of these cells to lysis via the alternate properdin pathway is under study by Rosse and his associates. One possibility is that the blood of patients with this disease contains several subpopulations of erythrocytes, some of which may possess the appropriate intermediates which lyse in the presence of acidified serum or merely by the addition of 0.6 m Eq/L (3 $\times$ 10^{-4} M) of magnesium. Indeed we have observed that magnesium itself can activate the properdin system. The validity of this hypothesis receives support from experiments conducted with cells of paroxysmal nocturnal hemoglobinuria patients treated with anti-I serum. This antibody is directed against the I antigen which is present on all human red cells. The number of C3 molecules bound to one of these cells increased from undetectable levels to 70, 121, and 192 upon the addition of magnesium, HCl, or both of these reagents, respectively. Rosse and others have found that PNH cells bind no more C4 than do normal erythrocytes. The greater susceptibility of PNH cells to lysis by an anti-I and C is attributable to an increased binding of C3, probably as C3b. As a result, a greater number of $C\overline{42}$ sites may be available on the PNH cells. Alternatively, the bound C3b on these cells could also promote activation of the alternate pathway, rendering even more C3b available for lysis of the cells through the feedback mechanism ascribed to C3b in this lytic pathway. It would seem, therefore, that hemolysis of PNH cells via the alternate pathway may be initiated by the early components of the classical pathway. When normal erythrocytes are present in reaction mixtures containing C activated by the properdin system, fluid-phase cleavage of C3 may proceed very rapidly together with conversion of C3b to its inactive form by KAF. On this basis, the formation of an active complex containing the immune aggregates, Factor B (C3PA), and other serum factors would not be productive in the lytic sequence. In contrast, the latter sequence does characterize the mechanism of erythrocyte lysis in the chain of reactions initiated with the cobra venom factor.

Cobra Venom Activation

The early studies of the marked anticomplementary action of cobra venom and, more specifically, its effect on C3 have been advanced with much success in recent years. Following the work of Klein and Wellensiek, and of Nelson who deprived guinea pigs of the C3 activity by parenteral injection of cobra venom, Müller-Eberhard and Fjellström isolated the active constituent and characterized it as a glycoprotein of β-mobility and with a molecular weight of 144,000. This achievement followed reports from several laboratories that a cobra venom factor (CVF) attacked the C system with a preferential destruction of C3 without the aid of antibody. The *in vivo* action of cobra venom seemed remarkably specific for C3 with little discernible effects on the formed elements of the blood or other serum constituents, save one. The purified CVF did not cleave C3 without the intervention of another serum factor, subsequently identified as Factor B (C3PA). Further investigations in other laboratories disclosed additional features of this reaction which mark the CVF-serum interaction as an alternate pathway which differs in several respects from the properdin system, thereby constituting a second alternate pathway. Some of its distinctive features are noted in Table 3-5.

The major differences between these two reaction mechanisms revolve about the participation of properdin and target cell lysis. Magnesium is an

Table 3–5

| | Activation of C by: | |
	Inulin, LPS, immune aggregates, etc.	Cobra venom factor
Properdin requirement	Essential	None
C3 requirement	Essential	Essential
C3PA (Factor B) requirement	Essential	Essential
C3PAse (Factor D) requirement	Essential	Essential
C3b feedback	Demonstrated	Unknown
Lysis of target cell	Not readily demonstrable	Readily demonstrable
Factor E requirement	Not readily demonstrable	Reported

essential cofactor as demonstrated by the Pillemer group for properdin and for the CVF pathway in our laboratory. We have also shown that heparin is an efficient inhibitor of the CVF mechanism, but neither the site of action nor its influence on the properdin system has been clarified.

The scheme outlined in Fig. 3-5 describes the current views of the sequence that is initiated upon the addition of CVF to fresh serum. Notable in this scheme is the indication based on the reports by Alper and co-workers that the union of CVF with C3PA requires the cooperation of at least one additional component, Factor D, originally identified as C3PAse

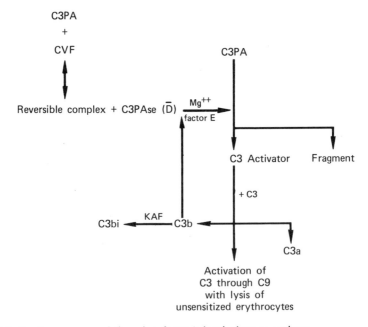

Fig. 3-5. Reaction sequence of the cobra factor induced alternate pathway.

or GBGAse. The role of Factor D in these events has been characterized by Cooper in the following terms. C3PA is considered to form a reversible complex with CVF with but a feeble capacity to effect the proteolysis of C3. In the presence of minute amounts of Factor D, this complex is stabilized and endowed with much greater efficiency for C3 cleavage. Reversible complex formation as a mechanism of C action has many precedents as discussed in the previous chapter. These include the loose association of gamma globulin with C1q, of C1q with C1r and C1s, C2 with C4, C5 with C6 and C7, and C8 with C9. This view has not yet gained universal acceptance since several investigators (Alper et al. and Hunsicker et al.) find that C3PA (Factor B) represents a serum component which is present in far lesser quantity than the amounts shown in Table 3-1, i.e., 100–200 μg per ml. The prevailing view tends to favor the data of Götze and Müller-Eberhard that C3PA is not a minor serum constituent, but this issue should soon be resolved. Mention must also be made of the report by Hunsicker and others that Factor E, an unidentified serum constituent, as well as C3PA and Factor D, are required to promote lysis of the unsensitized erythrocyte by CVF-treated serum.

These findings have been utilized in the author's laboratory for the construction of a two-step assay for estimating the level of Factor B in body fluids, an assay based on the hemolytic activity of this pathway. The fact that Factor B limits hemolysis in these assays is drawn from combined studies based on activity measurements in which the hemolytic potency of CVF-treated serum is correlated with immunochemical analyses with a monospecific antiserum carried out by Laurell's rocket immunoelectrophoresis procedure. As shown in Fig. 3-6, the amounts of C3PA, as judged by precipitation in gels, closely correspond to the degrees of lysis measured by the hemolytic assay. This assay expresses C3PA activity in terms of cobra venom activatable hemolysis, i.e., in $CVFH_{50}$ units, the reciprocal of the serum dilution which lyses 50% of a standardized suspension of erythrocytes following admixture of CVF with fresh serum. Since this assay has been used to study the biological activities of Factor B or C3PA, a brief description is in order. CVF is added in excess to a series of serum dilutions in a magnesium-fortified buffer. This step serves a double purpose. Incubation of this mixture leads to cleavage of all the C3 in the test serum and to the formation of the CVF·C3PA· Factor D complex and formation of the C3 Activator. In the second step, an excess of C3 as well as all the reagents needed to promote lysis are added in the form C-EDTA, i.e., guinea pig serum rendered 0.02 M with respect to EDTA. The presence of the chelating agent prevents further formation and/or activity of the CVF·C3PA·CD complex, so that the degree of hemolysis is directly proportional to the activity of C3PA in the test sample. A typical set of dose-response curves is shown in Fig. 3-7 taken from our studies.

Although most of the published studies with CVF have used the protein

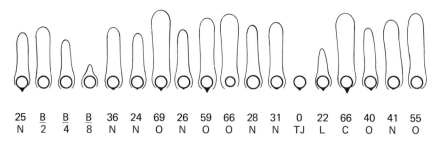

25	B	B	B	36	24	69	26	59	66	28	31	0	22	66	40	41	55
N	2	4	8	N	N	O	N	O	O	N	N	TJ	L	C	O	N	O

Fig. 3-6. Estimates of C3PA (Factor B) by Laurell's technique of immunoelectrophoresis. Mono-specific antibody was incorporated in the agar plate. Specimens were then added to the designated wells and electrophoresed. The numbers in the upper row represent the results of hemolytic assays of Factor B which correlate well with the precipitation area obtained for each specimen. The second, third, and fourth wells from the left, marked B, contained a purified preparation diluted 2-, 4-, and 8-fold. The specimen marked TJ was donated by Dr. Chester Alper. It was obtained from a patient whose serum lacked Factor B.

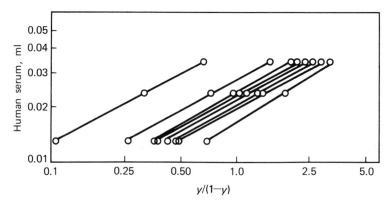

Fig. 3-7. Dose-response curves for lysis of E following CVF-serum interaction. The results obtained with sera from 8 different individuals are plotted according to the von Krogh equation, in which $y/(1-y)$ represents the degree of lysis. (From M. Brai and A. G. Osler, *P.S.E.B.M.*, **140**: 1116, 1972.)

isolated from the venom of *Naja naja* with human or guinea pig serum, the reaction is more general in nature. Other species may be employed as the source of CVF activities and of the C cofactors. Gewurz and his collaborators have found that the following sera may be substituted for human or guinea pig C: sera of embryonic, precolostral, newborn, and adult pig and cattle, as well as the sera of mice, rats, chickens, cobra, frog, and starfish. Rabbit serum is also an excellent reagent when used with guinea pig erythrocytes for C3PA assays of mouse sera.

The antibody-independence of these lytic reactions suggests that this

C-activation sequence represents a primordial host defense system which preceded the evolutionary development of specific immunoglobulins, as discussed in Chapter 5. The findings of Platts-Mills and Ishizaka are of interest in this context. They observed that fresh normal human serum lysed unsensitized rabbit erythrocytes in the presence of EGTA, and they attribute the lysis to activation of the alternate pathway in the absence of specific antibody. They speculate that this *in vitro* phenomenon involves an important recognition system for foreign antigens.

Other non-antibody mechanisms of C activation have been described which may not have physiological significance but whose mechanisms merit further investigation. The ability of silicic and tannic acids to replace the hemolytic antibody was mentioned in the previous chapter. Polyinosinic acid and several plasma and bacterial proteinases like streptokinase activate C1. The enzyme lysozyme forms a complex with single-stranded DNA which activates the entire C sequence. The interaction of several polyanions such as heparin, chondroitin sulfate, dextran sulfate, and hyaluronic acids with the polycations protamine, polybrene, or neomycin in fresh human serum leads to precipitate formation and C fixation. Preliminary studies indicate that these aggregates function by conversion of C1 to its esterolytic form as in the classical sequence. Continued study of these reactions may lead to a better definition of the nature of the C-activating sites than can be obtained with immune aggregates. May and Frank have observed that the alternate pathway may also be activated by sensitized sheep erythrocytes which have bound C1. Lysis of these cells requires about thirty times as much antibody as is needed for immune hemolysis through the classical sequence. Evidence for involvement of the alternate pathway was obtained in experiments showing that the EAC1 cells undergo destruction in sera lacking either C4, C2, or C6. Studies by Fearon and others indicate still another hemolytic route, i.e., the lysis of EAC43b in the presence of Factors **B** and **D**.

FURTHER READING

Alper, C. A., Goodkofsky, I., and Lepow, I. H., "The Relationship of Glycine-Rich β-Glycoprotein to Factor B in the Properdin System and to the Cobra Factor-Binding Protein of Human Serum," *J. Exp. Med.,* **137**:424, 1973.

Alper, C. A., and Rosen, F. S., "Genetic Aspects of the Complement System," *Adv. Immunol.,* **14**:251, 1971.

Brade, V., Lee, G., Nicholson, A., Shin, H. S., and Mayer, M. M., "The

Reaction of Zymosan with the Properdin System in Normal and C4-Deficient Guinea Pig Serum: Demonstration of C3- and C5-Cleaving Multi-Unit Enzymes," *J. Immunol.*, **111**:1389, 1973.

Brade, V., Nicholson, A., Lee, G., and Mayer, M. M., "The Reaction of Zymosan with the Properdin System: Isolation of Purified Factor D from Guinea Pig Serum and Study of its Reaction Characteristics," *J. Immunol*, **112**:1845, 1974.

Fearon, D. T., Austen, K. F., and Ruddy, S., "Properdin Factor D," *J. Exp. Med.*, **140**:426, 1974.

Fearon, D. T., Austen, K. F., and Ruddy, S., "Properdin Factor D: Characterization of its Active Site and Isolation of the Precursor Form," *J. Exp. Med.*, **139**:355, 1974.

Gewurz, H., Shin, H. S., and Mergenhagen, S. E., "Interactions of the Complement System with Endotoxic Lipopolysaccharides. Consumption of Each of the Six Terminal Complement Components," *J. Exp. Med.*, **128**:1049, 1968.

Götze, O., and Müller-Eberhard, H. J., "The C3-Activator System: An Alternate Pathway of Complement Activation," *J. Exp. Med.*, **134**:90s, 1971.

Götze, O., and Müller-Eberhard, H. J., "The Role of Properdin in the Alternate Pathway of Complement Activation," *J. Exp. Med.*, **139**:44, 1974.

Lepow, I. H., *The Properdin System: A Review of Current Concepts in Immunochemical Approaches to Problems in Microbiology*, M. Heidelberger and O. J. Plescia, eds., The Rutgers University Press, New Brunswick, N.J., 1961, p. 280.

Lew, F. T., Yukiyama, Y., Waks, H. S., and Osler, A. G., "Activation of the Alternative (Properdin) Pathway by Divalent Cations," *J. Immunol.*, in press.

Minta, J. O., and Lepow, I. H., "Studies on the Sub-Unit Structure of Human Properdin," *Immunochemistry*, **11**:361, 1974.

Müller-Eberhard, H. J., and Götze, O., "C3 Proactivator Convertase and its Mode of Action," *J. Exp. Med.*, **135**:1003, 1972.

Nelson, R. A., Jr., "An Alternative Mechanism for the Properdin System," *J. Exp. Med.*, **108**:515, 1958.

Nicholson, A., Brade, V., Lee, G., Shin, H. S., and Mayer, M. M., "Kinetic Studies of the Formation of the Properdin System Enzymes on Zymosan: Evidence That Nascent C3b Controls the Rate of Assembly," *J. Immunol.*, **112**:1115, 1974.

Osler, A. G., and Sandberg, A. L., "Alternate Complement Pathways," *Prog. in Allergy,* **17**:51, 1973.

Vallota, E. H., Götze, O., Spiegelberg, H. L., Forristal, J., West, C. D., and Müller-Eberhard, H. J., "A Serum Factor in Chronic Hypocomplementemic Nephritis Distinct from Immunoglobulins and Activating the Alternate Pathway of Complement," *J. Exp. Med.,* **139**:1249, 1974.

Chapter 4

Complement Fixation

The design of C-fixation reactions takes advantage of two major properties of C: the capacity to bind to immune complexes and to lyse sensitized cells. These two functions are separated in time by allowing the immune event under study to proceed in the presence of C and then testing for residual hemolytic capability with sensitized erythrocytes. This sequence, applied by Bordet and Gengou to the detection of antigens and antibodies, long represented the most widely used immunological reaction in the service of medicine, particularly as applied to the diagnosis of infectious diseases. The reaction is sensitive, specific, and can be performed with either soluble or particulate multivalent antigens that are not suitable for use in agglutination or specific precipitation tests. Complement fixation reactions have also been used for taxonomic purposes to establish immunochemical relationships among different antigens, to detect and estimate the quantity of specific antigens in body fluids (e.g., serum albumin in cerebrospinal fluid), for studies of antibody structure and functions, and for the detection of cell-bound macromolecules.

Complement fixation procedures can be classified into three categories. In the one most commonly used, the sensitized erythrocytes are added to the antigen-antibody-C reaction mixture upon completion of the latter reaction. A more quantitative procedure has been designed in which the amount of C remaining after termination of the first immune reaction is titrated to determine how much hemolytic activity was consumed by the immune system under study. More recently, Borsos and Rapp described C-fixation procedures for individual components which estimate the number of C1, C3, or C4 molecules bound by complexes formed on a cell surface or in the fluid phase. Before considering these methods in greater detail, we will discuss several properties of the reagents used in C-fixation reactions taking into account some of the newer developments. Readers interested in the technical aspects of this subject should consult the chapter by Mayer in Kabat and Mayer's *Experimental Immunochemistry* and the volume by Rapp and Borsos.

THE DOSE-RESPONSE CURVE IN IMMUNE HEMOLYSIS

As is widely known, this relationship is characterized by a sigmoid curve relating the degree of lysis to the volume of serum or the number of C units added to the sensitized erythrocytes, as shown in Fig. 4-1. The

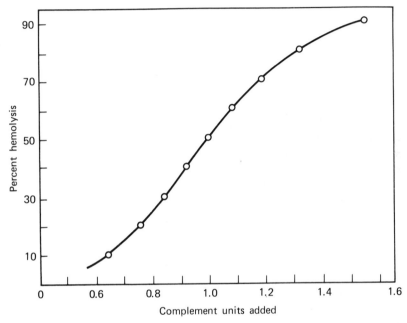

Fig. 4-1. Lysis of sheep erythrocytes sensitized with Forsmann antibody as a function of the amount of guinea pig C added. Based on a slope of 0.2 in the logarithmic transformation of von Krogh.

curve is essentially linear only in its central portion, indicating a decreased efficiency of the C system in the response ranges yielding less than 25% and more than 75% lysis. Our understanding of this sigmoid relationship has been considerably elucidated now that the individual components are available in purified form and their modes of action characterized. The initial lag in the curve may be attributed to several factors. The simplest interpretation, though not the most rigorous, is that one or more of the C components in the lower serum concentrations are not available in sufficient quantity to complete the entire lytic sequence.

Also as noted in Chapter 2, the C components do not function hemolytically with complete efficiency. In some instances, e.g., C4 and C2, there is considerable destruction in the fluid phase of reaction mixtures. The clustering effect of C4 and the binding of C3b to membrane sites which are not hemolytically productive also contribute to a lowered efficiency. There is still another plausible reason which stems from the fact that several of the reaction intermediates such as $\overline{EAC142}$ decay under the usual experimental conditions. If, then, the rate of decay of an intermediate exceeds the rate of utilization of the later components, the degree of lysis will not be proportional to the number of C units added, resulting in an initially delayed response. As more serum is added, the rates of decay and progression approach equality and the number of cells lysed is directly proportional to the amount of C added as is seen in the range of about 25 to 75% lysis. Thereafter, the slope declines again for the following reasons. Since it has been proven that immune lysis is a one-hit phenomenon, higher serum concentrations produce many redundant sites on the sensitized red cells which are no longer required for hemolysis. Moreover, the lysed red cell membranes are still capable of binding C components to build up nonhemolytic intermediates. As a result, the slope declines because the increments of C beyond the points needed to produce 75% lysis are even less efficient than those in the 25 to 75% range. The linear relationship in the latter range, coupled with the steeper slope of the dose-reaction curve, provided the rationale for introducing the 50% unit, CH_{50}, in preference to the titrations based on initial or complete lysis.

IMMUNOGLOBULIN CLASS AND C FIXATION

IgM

It is an intriguing fact that IgM antibodies formed early during the immune response in contrast to those of the IgG class are extremely efficient in activating the C sequence. In terms of specific activities based on weight units, the C-fixing potencies of the former immunoglobulins surpass those of the IgG class by several orders of magnitude. The basis for the heightened activity of the IgM antibodies may be due to their possession of ten combining groups, thereby facilitating the formation of a more complex matrix for binding C1q than is possible with their IgG counterparts. The macromolecular antibodies also have a higher mean affinity for antigen than do the IgG molecules synthesized during the early immune response. These factors may account for the observation that a single IgM molecule with Forssman antibody activity suffices to prepare an erythrocyte for lysis by C. A well-known laboratory observation is that rabbit antisera to boiled sheep stromata containing Forssman determinants are potent sensitizers provided the IgM:IgG ratio is elevated. Since non-C-fixing IgM antibodies have also been found, their presence will also govern the hemolytic activities of rabbit anti-Forssman sera. The feeble C-fixing potencies of early IgG immunoglobulins also have relevance for the study of antibody synthesis. Several years ago, we obtained sera from rabbits and guinea pigs during the first week after immunization with a single injection of human serum albumin. The 7S and 19S components were isolated by molecular sieve chromatography and the absolute antibody content of the two fractions was obtained by a modified antigen binding assay. The two immunoglobulin fractions were also assayed by several other procedures such as hemagglutination and passive cutaneous anaphylaxis. The results demonstrated that the 7S components were present in quantities exceeding those of the 19S constituents by molar ratios of 50 or more. Despite this fact, the 7S components were not demonstrable by several of the immunologic procedures based on secondary antibody properties such as C fixation and hemagglutination. The 19S immunoglobulins were about 500 times more active on a molar basis. The greater potency of the decavalent IgM as compared to the divalent IgG may also be referable to the disposition of the antigenic determinants on the cell membrane. Thus T. Ishizaka and her colleagues found that IgG and IgM human anti-blood group A substance were of comparable potency on a molar basis in C-fixation reactions carried out with soluble antigens. However, when the antigen was cell bound, as in the group A erythrocytes, the IgM immunoglobulins were more efficient. Plaut and collaborators have shown that IgM or its pentameric Fc fraction was far more efficient in reactions with human than with guinea pig C. This finding recalls the large body of work carried out by Christine Rice on the interchangeability of C and component mixtures with antisera of numerous species as noted in Chapter 2. Although these studies have found little application in recent years, they probably provide a sound starting point for future investigators.

IgG

The comparison of C-fixing potencies of IgM and IgG immunoglobulins has thus far failed to consider the parameter of heterogeneity within a single antibody class, a major variable for IgG immunoglobulins. As shown in Table 2-3, there are marked differences in this property among the four subclasses of human IgG insofar as the classical C system is concerned. It has recently been indicated that none of the human IgG subclasses can utilize the alternate pathway. This rather surprising observation was obtained when individual myeloma proteins aggregated by heat or treatment with bis-diazobenzidine were added to a human serum deficient in C2. It will be of some importance to confirm these findings with reaction systems that include human antibodies, rather than monoclonal proteins, in aggregates formed with specific antigens and with normal sera as a C source, to assure the availability of all the C reactants. The heterogeneity of guinea pig IgG immunoglobulins with respect to activation of the alternate and classical pathways has been discussed in Chapter 3. Similar differences between the IgG1 and IgG2 components have been observed in sera of rabbits, mice, and other species.

For many years, C-fixation tests have been used as a means of estimating the relative antibody content of different sera. The most widespread application has involved the use of early and convalescent sera in viral and other infections. The limitations of this procedure for such purposes were forcefully demonstrated in experiments with Wallace and others. Rabbit antisera to bovine serum albumin were obtained after one or two courses of immunization. Despite the intensity of immunization, which involved sixteen injections per course, there were marked differences in the C-fixing potencies of the sera expressed on a weight basis. The sera obtained after the second course were about four times more effective. Since the efficiency of C fixation, hemagglutination, and virus neutralization is modulated by the affinities of the immunoglobulins, it follows that an increase in titer may reflect this variable as well as an increment in antibody synthesis. The differences between IgM and IgG immunoglobulins in this respect further complicate the interpretations of C fixation titers in epidemiologic studies. These considerations stress the fact that C-fixation titers do not necessarily provide an accurate measure of antibody content. An illustrative experiment which is pertinent to the present discussion is summarized in Fig. 4-2. It may be seen that 5 μg of pneumococcal antibody N in the sera of three different rabbits show a sixfold variation in C-fixing ability in assays performed at 37° C with an input of 50 CH_{50}. These differences were less apparent when the fixation mixtures were carried out at 4° C with 50 CH_{50}. The role of antibody affinity in modulating these results has been demonstrated by Frank in a more dilute C-fixation system where differences in this property would be readily apparent. Sera with K_0 values ranging from 1.1 to 900 $\times$ 10^{-6} 1/mole yielded C-fixing antibody titers varying over a 15-fold range.

IgA

This immunoglobulin class, previously considered inert with respect to the C system, has recently been shown to activate the alternate pathway. In view of the concentration gradient established by these antibodies in close proximity to mucous membranes of the respiratory and intestinal tracts, interest has been heightened for the role of IgA in host defense mechanisms to bacterial and other infectious agents.

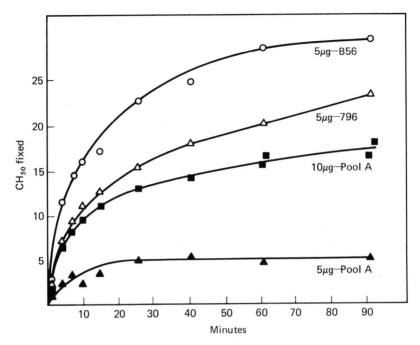

Fig. 4-2. C-fixing capacities of several rabbit anti-Pn III sera with SIII at equivalence zone ratios. Fixation-37°C in the presence of 50 CH_{50}. (From A. G. Osler and B. M. Hill, *J. Immunol.*, **75**: 143, 1955.)

IgE

These immunoglobulins, of primary concern in the release of vasoactive mediators like histamine and the slow-reacting substance of anaphylaxis (SRS-A), are feeble activators of the alternate pathway under *in vitro* conditions. Active sites have been detected in both the Fc piece and in the Fab dimer. These findings require further study in view of the relatively large quantities of the IgE myeloma aggregates used in these experiments.

The C-Fixing Sites on Immunoglobulin Molecules

Considerable effort has been devoted towards identifying the immunoglobulin regions that bind C1q in the classical pathway or activate the properdin sequence. Much of the earlier work was not readily interpretable because of the lack of awareness of the alternate pathway which resulted in wavering opinions as to the role of the $F(ab')_2$ fragment in C activation. The current views may be summarized as follows.

With respect to the classical pathway, it is now generally accepted, following the work of Amiraian, Taranta and their colleagues, that the Fc piece contains the binding site for C. The Ishizakas then demonstrated that aggregated Fc fragments are as potent as aggregated IgG preparations with respect to the fixation of C along the classical pathway, beginning with the binding of C1q. Attempts to localize the specific amino acid sequence within the Fc piece have been somewhat less productive since the three-dimensional structure of the molecule contributes substantially to its C-fixing capacity. Cleavage of the interchain disulfide bonds by reduction and alkylation or treatment with urea deprives the intact molecule of much of its C-fixing potential. Nevertheless, recent studies have pinpointed a sequence of about fifty amino acid residues within the hinge region of the IgG Fc piece as containing the active site. Two groups of investigators have isolated fragments obtained by controlled proteolysis of IgG and have studied their biologic activities. One such fragment, called H-5 by Kehoe and collaborators, contains about sixty amino acid residues. It possessed but 3% of the C-fixing potency of the Fc piece. This polypeptide was derived from the amino terminal half of the Fc region of a mouse IgG2a myeloma. Although these authors implicate C1q in this process, the fact that better fixation was obtained at $20°$ C rather than at $4°$ C suggests the possible involvement of the alternate pathway. Of interest is the finding that this 7,000 mol. wt. fragment is distal to the interchain disulfide bonds. Its location in the C_H2 domain indicates that the interchain disulfide does not participate in the fixation of C by this peptide.

Utsumi and his colleagues obtained quite different results in experiments with rabbit IgG. They isolated two papain digestion products of equivalent C-fixing potencies. In one, the Fc piece was still linked to an Fab fragment by a pair of labile disulfide bridges. The second C-activation site was located in the Fc piece which was released with an intact interchain bond. This fragment was also capable of skin fixation in the guinea pig, an essential step in mediating passive cutaneous anaphylaxis. The molecular weight of this fragment, 48,000, could be reduced by 2000 daltons with abrogation of skin fixation but without diminishing its C-fixing potency. Utsumi concluded that fixation of C by rabbit IgG requires a sequence of about fifty amino acids per heavy chain in a region near the amino terminus. Earlier, Prahl had shown that the C-terminal portion lacked biological activity.

The studies by Utsumi and by Kehoe and Fougereau were completed before the existence of alternate C pathways gained general recognition. As a result, it is not clear whether the sites discussed above could activate the classical or the alternate pathway. This uncertainty is strengthened by the realization that the C-fixation studies were performed with latex particles coated with the fragments. As seen in Chapter 3, preformed aggregates are efficient activators of the properdin pathway. Repetition of these experiments with component analyses would therefore be of considerable interest. Hurst and others recently studied the ability of the cyanogen bromide fragments of an IgM myeloma protein to bind $C\bar{1}$. A peptide containing only twenty-four amino acid residues on the amino terminal side of the disulfide loop making up the C_H4 domain possessed the $C\bar{1}$-fixing property.

Another interesting feature of C fixation by $F(ab')_2$ fragments, initially observed by Schur and Becker, emerges from a comparison of the dose-response curves generated by the untreated and pepsin-digested antibodies. An instructive illustration is given in Fig. 4-3 taken from the report by Reid.

As indicated, greater amounts of the $F(ab')_2$ fragments are required to initiate the reaction, and C fixation by these fragments is lesser in extent than that obtained with the intact antibody. These differences may be more apparent than real for the following reasons. As discussed previously, the factors limiting C fixation with IgG aggregates are referable to the decay of such intermediates as Ag.AbC1,4,2. As a consequence, the residual hemolytic activity in the reaction mixtures after completion of the fixation process is limited by a deficiency in the early-acting components. Other factors are at work with the $F(ab')_2$ fragments since the levels of C1, C4, and C2 do not govern alternate pathway activity. The limiting factor(s) here may be properdin, C3PAse (Factor D), C3PA (Factor B), or other components of this system. Consequently, a comparison of the C-fixing potencies of 7S and $F(ab')_2$ preparations may not be very meaningful when measured in terms of residual hemolytic activity by the classical system. The experiments of Schur and Becker support this interpretation. They found that fixation reaction mixtures set up with $F(ab')_2$ preparations rarely fixed more than about 40% of the available hemolytic activity. Supernates of these reaction mixtures could, however, serve as a C source for further fixation with the intact antibodies, clearly indicating that the two modes of C fixation were independent of each other: the one enters the alternate sequence at C3, while the 7S aggregates activate C1 as well as the properdin pathway.

The restriction that guinea pig IgG1 immunoglobulins and rabbit $F(ab')_2$ fragments interact with C through the alternate pathway may explain the inability of these antibodies to mediate passive immune hemolysis. For these experiments, unsensitized erythrocytes are coated with antigen and then incubated with C and specific antibody. The failure to observe lysis in these instances may be attributed to two factors. The first is the necessary use of diluted serum as a C source since higher concentrations often destroy the antigen-modified erythrocytes even in the absence of antibody. Undue dilution of the serum may favor one of the decay reactions at the sacrifice of the ongoing sequence necessary for cell destruction. In

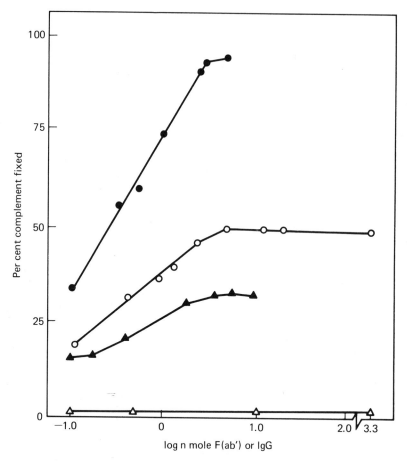

Fig. 4-3. The percentage of complement fixed is plotted against the logarithm of the antibody protein (in the form of preformed immune aggregates) present in the fixation mixture: ●, anti-HEA IgG 60 min at 37° or 18 hours at 4°; O, anti-HEA F(ab')$_2$ 60 min at 37°; ▲, anti-HSA (F(ab')$_2$ 60 min at 37°; △, anti-HEA F(ab')$_2$ 18 hours at 4°. (From K. B. M. Reid, *Immunology*, **20**: 652, 1971.) HEA = ovalbumin; HSA = human serum albumin.

addition, activation of the alternate pathway by immune aggregates, inulin, or zymosan does not result in cell lysis as discussed in Chapter 3. The negative findings obtained in these passive hemolysis studies cannot therefore be taken as evidence for the lack of C activation.

Let us now turn to an evaluation of the C-fixation procedures in current use, being aware that we have not yet considered the properties of the antigen in these reactions. These will emerge from the discussion of quantitative studies of C fixation.

THE CONVENTIONAL PROCEDURES

The C literature is replete with descriptions of C-fixation techniques based on the procedure originally described by Bordet and Gengou. The different methods share several features in common.

1. The sensitized erythrocytes are added after preliminary incubation of the antigen-antibody-C reaction mixtures.

2. The guinea pig serum used as a C source is diluted about 200-fold or more to yield one to five hemolytic units for potential uptake by the immune reactants under study.

3. The titer or C-fixing potency of the test serum is expressed as the dilution which, on admixture with a suitable and constant amount of antigen, consumes virtually all of the hemolytic C activity.

4. Comparative studies with different sera are expressed in terms of these endpoint titers.

Leaving detailed technical considerations aside, several other comments are pertinent. It is apparent that a valid C-fixation test requires careful standardization of all the reagents. To cite one example, the buffer used as diluent should supply adequate amounts of Ca^{++} and Mg^{++} for the full expression of C1 and C2 activities. The dilutions of antigen and antibody used in these assays should be selected so that their combined anticomplementary action will not consume substantial amounts of the available C. The experimental conditions must be poised to assure completion of the initial antigen-antibody reaction so that the residual C will be free to act on the EA without competition by the first-stage reactants. The demonstration that this condition is attainable is shown in Fig. 4-4.

Given optimal experimental conditions, the sensitivity of this reaction is such that subnanogram quantities of antigen or antibody from an intensively immunized individual can be readily detected. The threshold levels of these reactants may be further decreased with reductions in reaction volume, the number of target cells, and the amount of C available for the reaction. For these reasons there have been several successful attempts at scaling-down the reagent volumes and concentrations so as to heighten sensitivity.

MICRO-C-FIXATION METHOD

The procedure designed by Wasserman and Levine has been successful in this regard and has been used rather extensively for the detection and immunochemical characterization of antigens in the 0.1 ng range. This

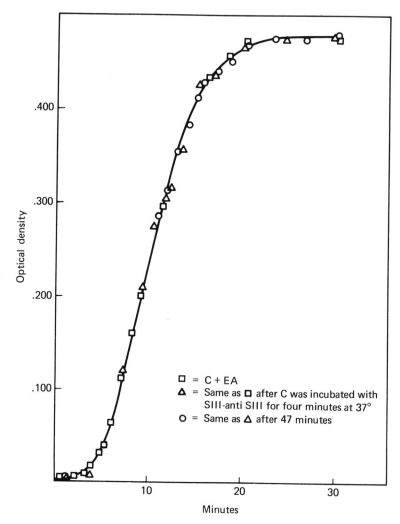

Fig. 4-4. Lack of competition for the hemolytic activity of C by sheep EA (□) and by rabbit anti-Type III pneumococcus serum plus SIII (△ and O). (From A. G. Osler and B. M. Hill, *J. Immunol.*, **75**: 141, 1955.)

micro-C-fixation technique employs 1.1 CH_{50}, 10^7 EA, and 3 ng of Forssman antibody N in a total volume of 0.7 ml, conditions which still permit spectrophotometric analyses of the liberated hemoglobin for the C titration and fixation assays. Even greater sensitivity has been attained in procedures based on the use of microtitrator plates and, in some cases, by the more laborious enumeration of the unlysed, residual cells, again with reduced volumes and target cell numbers.

Levine and his collaborators have used the micro procedure to great advantage in detecting antibody formation to nucleic acid derivatives in the sera of patients with systemic lupus erythematosus, in structural studies of many compounds, and in demonstrating the immunogenicity of a large variety of low molecular weight compounds with biological activities such as hormones, bradykinin, and angiotensin. In addition, inhibition studies of C fixation by monovalent haptens such as nucleotides and monosaccharides in Levine's laboratory have revealed important immunochemical relationships among related antigens based on their chemical composition and conformation. The reason for the heightened sensitivity of the Wasserman-Levine technique becomes apparent from an inspection of the curve of C lysis shown in Fig. 4-1. With an input of 1.1–1.2 CH_{50}, the maximum extent of lysis falls at about 70%. The slightest reduction in this value may be taken as evidence of an immune reaction, provided rigorous care is taken to show that all the procomplementary and anticomplementary controls are satisfactory. With an input of 1.2 CH_{50}, quantitation is restricted to the range of about 15–50% lysis or ca. 0.7 to 1.0 CH_{50}, and this is achieved by the use of appropriate dilutions of the antigen and antibody.

THE 5 CH_{50} UNIT METHOD

Similar reservations apply to procedures employing 5 CH_{50}. Here the limitations become apparent from the data in Table 4-1. In these systems,

Table 4–1

The relationships between the extent of hemolysis and the number of C units fixed in tests with an input of 5 CH_{50}

CH_{50} fixed	CH_{50} left	Percent lysis
None	5	100
1–3	2–4	100
4	1	50
5	0	0

partial hemolysis occurs only when 4 ± 0.5 CH_{50} are fixed. With greater or lesser fixation, lysis is either inapparent or complete, so that the immune reactants, usually the antiserum, is diluted to obtain lysis in the linear segment of the dose-response curve. As a result the reproducibility of this method is limited to a two-fold range.

Granted the convenience of these C-fixation procedures in performing large numbers of assays, some of the additional limitations require mention.

One which is common to all methods is that titrations of antisera based on C fixation provide only a relative estimate of the C-fixing activities in different sera, and not their total antibody content, for the reasons discussed earlier in this chapter. Moreover, methods based on the use of 1 or 5 CH_{50} are often not suitable for antibody detection since the high dilutions required to overcome anticomplementary effects restrict their use to antisera containing antibodies of relatively high affinity. Those with low avidity will not form sufficiently stable immune complexes to activate the C system. Another restriction stems from the fact that immune complexes whose ability to utilize C is limited to the alternate pathway will escape detection because the components of this C system are not functional when the concentration of the serum used as a C source falls below 5%, as indicated in Table 3-3. A notable example of this failure occurred in studies with the IgG2 guinea pig immunoglobulins. When hyperimmune reference antisera are employed to detect or compare the immunologic reactivity of different antigenic determinants, the methods based on five or fewer CH_{50} have been used with great success.

QUANTITATIVE C FIXATION

A partial means of resolving these limitations became available through the design of a quantitative C-fixation technique based on spectrophotometric assays of hemolytic C activity. This method departs from the conventional procedures in that the C input is increased from 5 CH_{50} to 50, 100, or 200 units. The antigen-antibody reaction is adjusted so that only a fraction of the available C is consumed. The method therefore involves two C titrations, one to determine the input and the second to estimate the number of hemolytic units remaining after completion of the immune reaction. The difference in the two values indicates the C-fixing potency of the immune system under study. Both titrations follow similar dose-response curves if the experimental conditions are adjusted to leave substantial C activity available for the second titration with sensitized erythrocytes.

Experiments carried out with a constant amount of antigen and antibody and varying amounts of guinea pig C show that the number of CH_{50} units fixed increases with greater amounts of available C. In a typical experiment, the interaction of 50, 100, and 200 CH_{50} units with the same quantity of antigen and antibody at 37° C resulted in the inactivation of 27, 34, and 52 CH_{50}, respectively. Extrapolation of these findings to *in vivo* conditions, wherein the immune reactants are in contact with vastly more C for longer periods of time, would lead one to expect even more intense fixation in terms of C units. Conversely, and as already indicated, the failure to observe C fixation in the presence of 5 CH_{50} does not exclude a role for C under *in vivo* conditions, a deduction unfortunately drawn in some studies of pathogenetic mechanisms. On the other hand, the demonstration of C fixation is but an initial clue that requires additional investigation before an essential role for C can be deduced.

PROPERTIES OF THE IMMUNE COMPLEX WITH C-FIXING ABILITY

The quantitative C-fixation studies provided definitive evidence that, for a constant amount of antibody, the extent of fixation may vary markedly with the quantity of antigen. The data in Fig. 4-5 exemplify this statement for the immune systems involving a constant quantity of rabbit antibodies reacting with either a polysaccharide or a protein antigen. It is clear that the shape of the quantitative C-fixation curve parallels that of specific precipitation at antibody levels which are only a minute fraction of that required to yield visible aggregation.

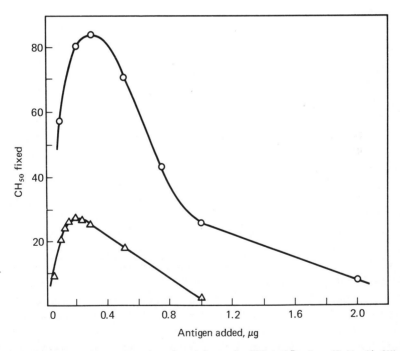

Fig. 4-5. Fixation of guinea pig C by: △ : 1.9 μg of rabbit anti-Pn. Type III N with SIII at 37°C for 60 min. C added: 50 CH_{50}. O : 1.8 μg of rabbit anti-duck egg albumin N with duck egg albumin at 4°C overnight. C added: 100 CH_{50}

As the data in Fig. 4-5 show, the degree of fixation rises steeply as the antigen:antibody ratio approaches equivalence as defined for specific precipitation. When more antigen is added, fixation of C decreases, approaching a value of zero at a ratio approximating two, in complete accordance with the course of precipitation. Since polysaccharides are polydisperse, transformation of these weight ratios into molecular terms is not feasible. However, studies with ovalbumin and other protein immune systems showed that complexes formed in extreme antigen excess, i.e., with the molecular composition of Ag_2Ab, fail to activate the C system. This conclusion was strengthened several years later by the Ishizakas who characterized the complexes in physicochemical terms and found that immune fixation of C required the close apposition of at least two antibody molecules, a condition fulfilled by aggregates of the composition Ag_3Ab_2 and preferably those even further enriched with antibody. These investigators also showed that the antigens were dispensable in endowing gamma globulin molecules with C-fixing properties. Aggregation of gamma globulin by gentle heating ($63°$ C, 20 min) or by treatment with bisdiazobenzidine produced complexes whose C-fixing potencies were on a par with those formed by interaction with antigen.

The C-fixation studies described in Fig. 4-5 and their extension by the Ishizakas provided experimental support for the postulate offered earlier by Heidelberger to the effect that C, probably C1, formed a loose, dissociable union with gamma globulin that was more firmly established by the three-dimensional lattice of multivalent antigen and antibody. The need for multivalency to form these lattices for the fixation of C is now universally accepted.

The multivalent antigen requirement is firmly based on evidence derived from inhibition experiments with haptens, while the role of bivalent antibody has emerged from two approaches. Fixation of C is inhibited by monomer Fab antibody fragments capable of binding only single antigen molecules. An additional demonstration emerged from the use of reconstituted, hybrid antibody molecules. Rabbit IgG dissociates into two half-molecules consisting of one light and one heavy chain after mild reduction at pH 5 and subsequent acidification to pH 2.5. These half-molecules do not fix C. On restoring the pH to neutral values, the half-molecules recombine to form a product with immunochemical properties similar to the native IgG molecules which are capable of precipitating the homologous antigen and activating the C system. When half-molecules of anti-ovalbumin are reconstituted in the presence of half-molecules of normal IgG, the product inhibits both specific precipitation of the antigen and of C-fixation in the reaction between ovalbumin and intact anti-ovalbumin IgG. The hybrid molecules in concentrations 100 times greater than the amounts of the native antibody fail to react. It is apparent that the C-fixing activity of antibody requires that both combining sites of the molecule must react with a multivalent antigen to initiate specific aggregate formation and C-fixation. This question has received renewed attention in the studies of Cohen and of Hyslop, Dourmashkin, Green, and Porter. Cohen's conclusions are consistent with the earlier studies in identifying the minimal C-fixing complex as one containing two adjacent antibody molecules linked by a multivalent antigen. The latter group reached a different conclusion from the results of experiments with purified antibodies and the divalent hapten bis-dinitrophenyl octamethylene diamine, reagents which permitted better characterization of the antibody-hapten complexes. The conclusion that complexes composed of tetramers and pentamers were more efficient than dimers and trimers in initiating C fixation may not conflict with deductions drawn from studies with the more complex antigens. Electron microscopic studies by Hyslop and others showed that the angle between the Fab arms of each IgG molecule lay between 90° and 180° in the active complexes. This angle was less than 60° in the inactive complexes. On this basis it may be inferred that adequate spreading of the Fab arms occurs during the interaction of two adjacent bivalent IgG antibody molecules with randomly spaced dissimilar determinants on multivalent antigens. With the chemically defined haptens containing two identical determinants in a closer spatial relationship, the union with four or five IgG molecules was required to attain the molecular architecture required to yield the same degree of C fixation. Another factor to be considered in the experiments of Hyslop et al. is the inability of the smaller complexes to activate the alternate pathway in the highly diluted reaction systems used by these investigators. While their results are applicable to C1q binding with activation of the classical system, it would be of interest to assess the capacity of the dimers and trimers to cleave C3 in undiluted serum via the alternate pathway.

The biologic activities manifested by aggregated gamma globulins have been taken into account in the clinical use of these proteins for passive immunization. Removal of these aggregates is now practiced routinely in preparing gamma globulin solutions for prophylactic use in viral and other infections with a concomitant reduction in the incidence of unfavorable side reactions.

A note of dissent regarding the need for multivalency and aggregation of antibody in C fixation has recently been entered by Plaut and co-workers. They found that the Fc portion of the IgM pentamer had the greatest efficiency for C fixation but the Fc monomers were also active. The explanation for this finding may perhaps be related to the spatial distribution of the immunoglobulin binding site on the monomeric preparation, but it is apparent that further work is needed to clarify the interpretation of this finding. Parenthetically, these immunoglobulins and their fractions fixed human C but not that of the guinea pig. Further study of these interesting findings are needed to reconcile this report with that of Hyslop and co-workers who failed to observe fixation of C by single molecules of IgM unless they were bound to antigen.

THE NATURE OF THE ANTIGEN AS A DETERMINANT OF C FIXATION

Several investigators have reported marked variations in the efficiency and temperature dependence of C fixation with respect to the nature of the antigen. A summary of relevant findings is given in Table 4-2.

Table 4–2 *

| | | | Relative extent of CF with: | | |
| | | | Whole serum | 19S | 7S |
Serum	Antigen	Fixation temperature	% fixation		
Rabbit anti-lipopolysaccharide	Colicin K	4	3600 †	800	1920
		37	2650	2300	<20 ‡
Human lupus erythematosus	Denatured DNA	4	<20		
		37	295	210	75
Human syphilis	Cardiolipin	4	3600	610	1430
		37	960	550	110
Rabbit anti-KLH (keyhole limpet hemocyanin)	KLH	4	410	<20	250
		37	<20	<20	<20

* Modified from, R. V. Cunniff and B. D. Stollar, J. Immunol., 100:9, 1968.
† Number refers to serum dilution yielding maximal C fixation.
‡ Less than 20% fixation at a serum dilution of 1:100 or less.

Several comments are noteworthy in the interpretation of these data. Since highly dilute C-fixation reaction mixtures were used (technique of Wasserman and Levine), the titers probably reflect only the activities of high-affinity antibodies. Moreover, a comparison of titers obtained with the 19S and 7S immunoglobulins at the same fixation temperature is not informative unless the fixation titers are expressed in terms of specific activities, i.e., the number of CH_{50} units fixed per mg of antibody. The available data indicate that the weight-specific potency of the 19S immunoglobulins may exceed that of the 7S molecules derived from the same serum sample by several orders of magnitude. The variation in results obtained with the same immune system at the two temperatures may be due in part to differences in the efficiency of activating the classical and alternate pathways, particularly in view of the temperature dependence of the latter, as shown in Chapter 3. Studies of this type with the 7S immunoglobulins are best performed separately with the gamma-1 and gamma-2 components in the light of their divergent behavior with the two C-activation systems.

ANTIGEN ASSAYS BY C FIXATION

The fixation of C provides a sensitive means for the estimation and characterization of antigens based on the availability of a calibration curve obtained with varying amounts of antigen and an excess of antibody. The data in Fig. 4-6 illustrate one application in which a potent rabbit anti-

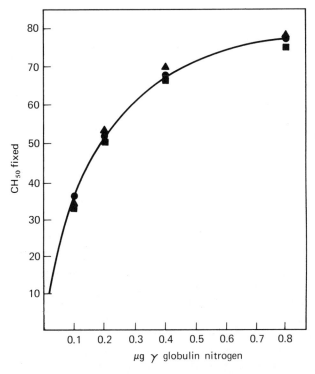

Fixation of guinea pig C at 4°C—20 hrs
Antibody: 3.0 μg Ra-Anti human γ globulin N
Antigen: Human γ globulin

CH$_{50}$ fixed

μg γ globulin nitrogen

Fig. 4-6. Calibration curve for estimating the amount of human gamma globulin bound by calf thymus nucleoprotein in sera of patients with systemic lupus erythematosus. ● , ■ , ▲ : Results of replicate experiments. (From A. S. Townes, C. R. Stewart, and A. G. Osler, *Bull. Johns Hopkins Hospital*, **112:** 186, 1963.)

serum to human gamma globulin was used to construct a reference curve for estimating the level of antinucleoprotein antibodies capable of specific binding to calf thymus nucleoprotein, a useful measure of the disease-associated immune response in the sera of patients with systemic lupus erythematosus. Many similar examples may be drawn from the reports of Levine and his collaborators.

Another application, in which quantitative C fixation has been used for the immunochemical characterization of phospholipid antigens, is described in Fig. 4-7. In this and other experiments, the sera of human

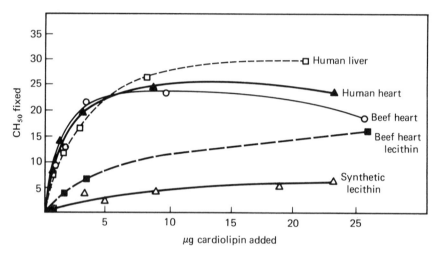

Fig. 4-7. Fixation of complement by human syphilis serum (1333) with human liver, human heart, and beef heart cardiolipins plus synthetic lecithin, and with beef heart and synthetic lecithins in the absence of cardiolipin. (From A. G. Osler and E. A. Knipp, *J. Immunol.,* **78**: 38, 1957.)

syphilis patients failed to distinguish between cardiolipins derived from human or bovine tissues. The C-fixation curves were virtually superimposable for the human and bovine Wassermann antigens, thereby providing a theoretical justification for the long-standing empirical use of beef heart extracts in serologic studies of this disease.

Prager and Wilson have provided an instructive demonstration of the usefulness of C fixation in studying immunologic and taxonomic relationships among a group of related antigens. Their experiments also reinforce the identity of reaction mechanisms in specific precipitation and C fixation. As antigens, they used purified lysozymes isolated from seven species of birds and showed that the extent of cross-reactivity of these enzymes with heterologous antisera was based on the number of differences in the amino acids sequences. The cross reactions, measured by means of quantitative precipitation and double diffusion were quantitatively similar. They then compared these differences with those obtained by microcomplement fixation employing the latter at almost 1000-fold lower concentrations, and their results are plotted in Fig. 4-8.

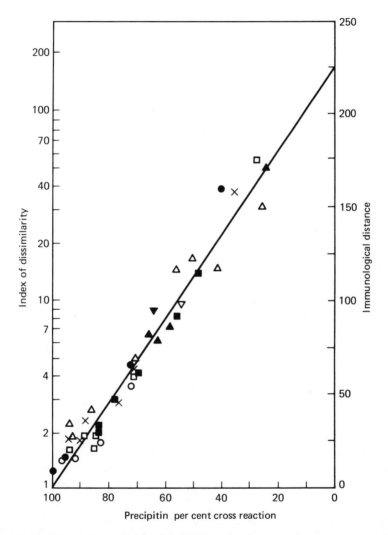

Fig. 4-8. Antigenic differences as measured by cross-reaction in the quantitative precipitin test (horizontal axis) and in the quantitative micro-complement fixation test (vertical axis). The tests were carried out with the following antisera: anti-chicken Pools 4 (●) and 6 (O); anti-bob-white quail Pool 6 (X); anti-turkey Pool 6 (□); anti-Japanese quail Pool 6 (△); anti-Duck A Pools 2 (▽), 4 (▼), and 6 (▲); and anti-ring-necked pheasant Pool 6 (■). (From E. M. Prager and A. C. Wilson, J. Biol. Chem., 246: 7012, 1971.)

It is readily apparent that the micro-C-fixation reactions characterized the antigenic differences quantitatively to the same extent as did the precipitin reactions at much higher concentrations of the immune reactants. It should be noted that the antisera used in these experiments were obtained after intensive immunization of the birds so as to obtain reagents suitable for the detection and quantitation of the cross reactions.

$\overline{CI}$ Fixation and Transfer Test

In 1965 Borsos and Rapp described a novel C-fixation assay, the $\overline{CI}FT$, applicable to measuring the number of C1 molecules bound by antigen-antibody complexes. The method is based on the binding property of C1 to aggregated immunoglobulins at low ionic strength ($\mu = 0.065$) and its quantitative dissociation and subsequent attachment to EAC4 at isotonicity ($\mu = 0.15$). As described by these investigators, the procedure is operationally divisible into three steps:

1. Fixation: $\text{Ag Ab} + \overline{CI} \xrightarrow{\mu = 0.065} \text{Ag Ab } \overline{CI} + \overline{CI}$

2. Transfer: $\text{Ag Ab } \overline{CI} + \text{EAC4} \xrightarrow{\mu = 0.15} \text{EAC}\overline{I}4 + \text{Ag Ab}$

3. Lysis: $\text{EAC}\overline{I}4 + \text{C2} + \text{C-EDTA} \rightarrow \text{hemolysis}$

This procedure can be modified for use with non-C-fixing immunoglobulins by treating these complexes with an anti-antibody reagent. The inability of guinea pig IgG1 to fix C1 was demonstrated with these techniques. The $\overline{CI}FT$ procedure has had several important applications.

Detection of Antigens on Cell Surfaces

The maximum uptake of $\overline{CI}$ by human chronic lymphocytic leukemia cells and a rabbit antiserum corresponded to about 7×10^4 molecules of $\overline{CI}$ per cell. Use of this method has also demonstrated that the number of virus-induced antigenic determinants per cell ranges from 50 to 600, while the number of IgM anti-Forssman antibody molecules capable of erythrocyte binding has been estimated at 7×10^4. Shortly after these studies were reported, it was shown that rabbit IgG hemolysins are not suitable for titrations of C1 on a molecular basis in human or guinea pig serum. This conclusion was based on the finding that, while IgG and IgM both fixed C1 to a roughly equivalent extent, the macromolecular immunoglobulin was far more active in converting C1 to $\overline{CI}$ on EAC4. In addition, use of the IgG antibodies leads to an overestimation of the number of $\overline{CI}$

molecules in sera because these immunoglobulins tend to transfer from site to site even at low ionic strength.

Comparative C-fixation Potencies of 7S and 19S Immunoglobulins

In another illustration, the 19S and 7S antibody classes were separated from a rabbit anti-ovalbumin serum. The antigen was coupled to human erythrocytes and the cells reacted with several dilutions of the antibody preparations. $\overline{\text{CIFT}}$ assays with these cells showed that the slope of the dose-response curves obtained with the 7S immunoglobulins was about twice that for the 19S antibodies. The illustrative data are given in Fig. 4-9. Interesting data pertaining to the temperature dependency of C fixation

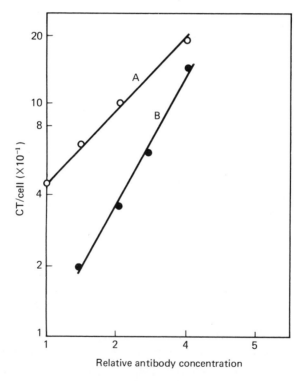

Fig. 4-9. $\overline{\text{CIFT}}$ by rabbit 19 S and 7 S anti-ovalbumin antibodies. Antiserum: commercial hyperimmune rabbit anti-ovalbumin serum. The serum was fractionated on Sephadex G 200. Curve A: dose-response curve with antibodies contained in the most excluded proteins ("19 S"); Curve B: dose-response curve obtained with antibodies contained in the intermediate protein peak ("7 S"). Antigen: reagent grade ovalbumin coupled to human B^+ cells by 1-ethyl-3-(3-dimethylaminopropyl) carbodiimide HCl. (From T. Borsos et al., *J. Immunol.*, **101**: 394, 1968.)

by 7S and 19S immunoglobulins have been obtained with $\overline{\text{C1}}$FT as shown in Table 4-3.

Table 4–3

Effect of temperature on $\overline{\text{C1}}$ fixation by sheep RBC-Forssman antibody complexes *

Temperature of fixation, °C	$\overline{\text{C1}}$FT sites per cell	
	7S	19S
0	380	30
13	120	40
25	30	100
37	0	120

* From T. Borsos et al., J. Immunol., **101**:396, 1968.

The $\overline{\text{C1}}$FT test has also been used to resolve the problem of C fixation with chicken antisera. These reagents do not react with guinea pig $\overline{\text{C1}}$ and are inconvenient to use because of their pronounced anticomplementary activities, particularly after inactivation. Stolfi and colleagues circumvented this problem by developing a $\overline{\text{C1}}$FT with chicken $\overline{\text{C1}}$. The use of the $\overline{\text{C1}}$FT has thus been extended and is now available for studies of virus diseases in fowls.

An application of the $\overline{\text{C1}}$FT procedure to the solution of biological problems has recently been described by Dr. Teruko Ishizaka and her associates. Using basophil-rich suspensions (10 to 40% basophils) prepared from peripheral blood, they estimated that cells furnished by allergic donors contained 15,000 to 41,000 molecules of IgE per basophil as compared to 4000 to 27,000 sites per basophil in blood furnished by normal controls. Since these levels did not correlate well with histamine release by a monospecific rabbit antiserum to IgE, they suggested that both the number and affinity of the basophil-bound IgE rather than IgE serum levels governed the histamine release response to the allergenic antigen. An additional interpretation to be considered is the binding of $\overline{\text{C1}}$ to cell-bound C4 sites which are not hemolytically productive (see Chapter 2). As a result of the clustering effect, to cite but one example, the binding of $\overline{\text{C1}}$ may be amplified without any pertinent physiologic significance. The association constant of the IgE-basophil interaction was estimated at 10^8 to 10^9 l/mole. The number of receptors was increased 2- to 6-fold with cells from atopic individuals and 1.1- to 2.0-fold with cells from normal controls. These studies also revealed that the number of IgE molecules per cell as well as biochemical factors operative after cell binding were important parameters for the release of histamine from basophils. Finally, they corroborated the earlier experiments of Dr. A. Secchi in our laboratory that basophils also bind IgG, albeit in a somewhat different distribution pattern. However, the release of histamine resulting from the IgG-antigen interaction does not seem to be an important event in this allergic reaction.

Estimation of C3

Borsos and Leonard have recently described a useful procedure for determining the amount of C3 or C3b bound to a cell membrane or in various body fluids. The amount of C3 in the test material is estimated by its addition to a reference quantity of C3 antiserum. The residual anti-C3 content is then assayed with EC3 indicator cells which lyse in the presence of guinea pig serum. Comparison of the degree of lysis thus obtained with the inhibition of lysis in the presence of a standard amount of C3 provides a measure of the C3 content of the material under study. Alternatively, the amount of cell-bound C3 can be determined by the $\overline{CI}$ fixation and transfer test with the use of a C3 antiserum. The reaction sequence used in these procedures is outlined in Table 4–4. As shown in this table, the cells are

Table 4–4

Fixation of human C3 to sheep erythrocytes *

Step	Reaction		Product
1	E + IgM	→	EAIgM
2	EAIgM + diluted human serum	→	EAIgMC3
3	EAIgMC3 + 2-mercaptoethanol	→	EC3
4	EC3 + anti-C3	→	EC3-anti-C3
5	EC3-anti-C3 + C	→	lysis, or as an alternative
6	EC3-anti-C3 + $\overline{CI}$	→	EC3-anti-C3-$\overline{CI}$
7	EC3 + anti-C3-$\overline{CI}$ + C4 + C5 through C9	→	lysis

* From T. Borsos and E. J. Leonard, *J. Immunol.*, **107**:767, 1971.

sensitized in step 1 and incubated with human serum in step 2 to yield cell-bound C3. The antibody is removed in step 3 and the product, EC3, is treated with a specific antiserum. The addition of C results in lysis; so the amount of C3 present in the sample used in step 2 can be estimated directly or with the aid of the $\overline{CI}$FT. In the former instance, fluid-phase C3 or C3 bound to other complexes will inhibit lysis, thereby providing a means of estimating cell-bound C3 by virtue of its inhibitory capacity. An illustration of the inhibition-of-lysis assay for C3 bound to Sepharose beads is given in Fig. 4-10.

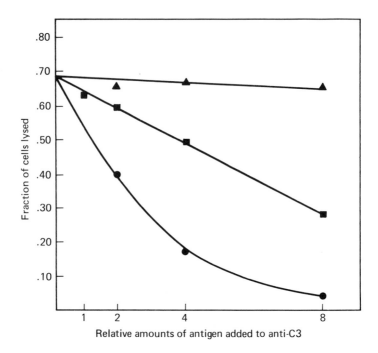

Fig. 4-10. Inhibition of lysis assay for C3 on Sepharose beads. Antigens include EC3 (■), Sepharose-albumin immune complex incubated with human serum (●) and the same in the presence of 0.01M EDTA (▲). From T. Borsos and E. J. Leonard, *J. Immunol.*, **107**: 770, 1971.

A limitation of the assay based on absorption of the anti-C3 by the test serum emerges from the fact that inactivated C3 contains several different antigenic determinants, not all of which are equally accessible to interaction with the standard antiserum. Nevertheless the method should prove useful in studies designed to implicate C, and more specifically C3, in studies of neoplastic or other immunopathologic situations.

An entirely analogous procedure for the immunochemical quantitation of cell-bound C4 was recently described by Ohanian and Borsos. The use of this inhibitor-of-lysis procedure indicated that the average C4 content of human sera was 718 ± 61 μg per ml. The value for a pool of guinea pig sera based on quantitative precipitin assays was 1106 ± 106 μg per ml.

IMMUNE ADHERENCE

About twenty years ago (and later in collaboration with D. S. Nelson), R. A. Nelson, Jr. explored the mechanism of another type of C fixation, immune adherence. This reaction emphasizes the capacity of C to induce the attachment of sensitized soluble or particulate antigens to adhere to primate erythrocytes or nonprimate platelets. Rosse and others have shown that red cells with membrane-bound C3 will adhere to granulocytes in the absence of antibody. The reaction is C and temperature-dependent and has been widely applied to the detection and estimation of antigens, antibodies, or C3. Measurements are made by hemagglutination or microscopic observation of the cell-bound aggregates. The requirement for C3 was established by Nishioka and Linscott, who demonstrated that the active intermediate contained the components C4 and C3. The formation of these C intermediates with immune aggregates is thought to promote immune clearance and phagocytosis.

In view of the high concentration of C3 in mammalian sera (e.g., guinea pig and human) and the dependence of immune adherence on C3, this reaction can be performed with smaller amounts of these sera than are required for immune hemolysis. Thus, although guinea pig serum is more efficient than human serum in immune hemolysis (ratio = 6), they are equipotent in immune adherence with immune complexes containing such antigens as sheep erythrocytes, Salmonella organisms, *Brucella abortus,* bacteriophage T2, serum albumins, etc. An indication as to the sensitivity of immune adherence reaction is given by R. A. Nelson, Jr. in a comparison of the reactivities of different rabbit anti-erythrocyte sera in several immunologic assays. Studies of five sera with antibody contents ranging from 0.39 to 0.62 mg N per ml yielded the following range of titers for:

1. Hemolysis	4800	to	38,000
2. Agglutination	1600	to	8000
3. Phagocytosis	2700	to	11,000
4. Immune adherence	96,000	to	780,000

Activation of the alternate pathway in C4-deficient guinea pigs by lipopolysaccharides and immune complexes has also been used to demonstrate immune adherence.

Complement Fixation by Protein A from Staphylococcus Aureus

In 1966 Forsgren and Sjöquist isolated a cell-wall constituent from a strain of a coagulase-producing *Staph. aureus.* This substance, Protein A, of molecular weight 42,000 possessed the capacity of precipitating IgG, a property originally attributed to natural antibodies in IgG preparations. Later studies showed that the precipitation occurred through interaction of Protein A with the Fc portion of the IgG molecule and not through the antibody combining groups. This finding led to the demonstration that the

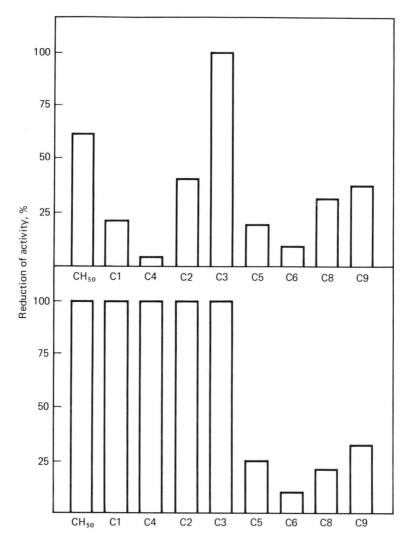

Fig. 4-11. Reduction of the activity of total complement and complement components in human serum after incubation with protein A and with preformed complexes between protein A and fragment Fc from IgG1. 200 μl aliquots containing (a) 200 μg of protein A; (b) preformed complexes, obtained by incubating 200 μg of protein A with 2 mg of Fc, were incubated with 1 ml of human serum for 60 min. at 37°C. The activities were measured hemolytically. Depletion of more than 98 per cent of the activity is depicted as 100 per cent depletion in the diagram. From G. Stålenheim et al., *Immunochemistry,* **10**: 504, 1973.

Protein A-IgG complex activated the C system with consumption of its hemolytic potential, thereby clarifying one of the invasive mechanisms associated with these pathogenic bacteria. This reaction which reduces the cytocidal and phagocytic capacities of the host may well provide a model for studying the invasiveness of other infectious organisms, particularly since the products of C activation may be destructive to the neighboring tissues.

Mixtures of Protein A and human serum fixed C more effectively at 37° C than at 4° C. At the higher temperature, the course of C fixation, for a constant amount of IgG and increasing Protein A, resembled that obtained with antigen and antibody. A profile of component consumption produced by incubating 200 μl aliquots of human serum with Protein A is depicted in Fig. 4-11. As may be noted, virtually all of the C3 activity was depleted by these complexes, with but minimal consumption of C4, unless preformed aggregates were used. Neither C4 nor C2, when added alone and in purified form to Protein A, were reduced in activity. Evidence for the participation of the alternate pathway was readily obtained in experiments showing a 40–60% activity loss of C3PA in reaction mixtures containing human serum and Protein A. Similar dose-response curves for C consumption by Protein A were observed for both the classical and alternate pathways. Since protein A inhibited the binding of $C\overline{1}$ by an IgG1 myeloma protein or its Fc fragment, it was concluded that the activation site for $C\overline{1}$ and the binding site for Protein A are close to each other on the immunoglobulin molecule. Two biologic consequences have already been shown to follow the Protein A-serum interaction, C-dependent platelet injury, and chemotaxis of polymorphonuclear leukocytes, the latter occurring with but a few micrograms of the staphylococcal product.

FURTHER READING

Borsos, T., Colten, H. R., Spalter, J. S., Rogentine, N., and Rapp, H. J., "The C′1a Fixation and Transfer Test," *J. Immunol.,* **101**:392, 1968.

Borsos, T., and Leonard, E. J., "Detection of Bound C3 by a New Immunochemical Method," *J. Immunol.,* **107**:766, 1971.

Levine, L., "Determinants of Specificity of Proteins, Nucleic Acids and Polypeptides," *Federation Proc.,* **21**:711, 1962.

Logue, G. L., Rosse, W. F., and Adams, J. P., "Complement-Dependent Immune Adherence Measured with Human Granulocytes," *Clin. Immunol. and Immunopathology,* **1**:398, 1973.

Mayer, M. M., "Complement and Complement Fixation," Chapter 4, in Kabat and Mayer's *Experimental Immunochemistry,* C. C. Thomas, Springfield, Ill., 1961.

Osler, A. G., "Quantitative Studies of Complement Fixation," *Bact. Revs.* **22**:246, 1958.

Prager, E. M., and Wilson, A. C., "The Dependence of Immunological Cross-Reactivity upon Sequence Resemblance among Lysozymes," *J. Biol. Chem.*, **246**:7010, 1971.

Rapp, H. J., and Borsos, T., *Molecular Basis of Complement Action*, Appleton-Century-Crofts, New York, 1970.

Stålenheim, G., Götze, O., Cooper, N. R., Sjöquist, J., and Müller-Eberhard, H. J., "Consumption of Human Complement Components by Complexes of IgG with Protein A of *Staphylococcus aureus*," *Immunochemistry*, **10**:501, 1973.

Chapter 5

Developmental Aspects
of the Complement System

Although immunologists have been greatly concerned with the biochemistry and phenomenology of the C system, relatively little effort has been expended in developmental studies. Yet there is little doubt but that our understanding of the evolutionary development of these highly complex reaction systems, which may have preceded antibody formation, is essential for a full appreciation of the role of C in the host's economy. Now that many of the individual components and their monospecific antisera are available, a considerable spurt of studies may be anticipated which will attempt to delineate the evolutionary and ontogenetic development of the complement system.

ONTOGENY AND BIOSYNTHESIS

Data pertaining to the ontogenetic development of hemolytic C activity are available for several species. Synthesis of C components has been demonstrated in chick embryos where maternal transmission can be excluded. Gabrielsen and her co-workers provided data to show that detectable hemolytic activity is demonstrable in the chick embryo and rises sharply within the first week after hatching as shown in Fig. 5-1. Activity levels of C1 follow a substantially similar course. Microbial colonization in chicken tissues seemingly has no effect on hemolytic C titers which are entirely comparable in animals bred in a conventional or germ-free environment.

Fetal sera of cattle and sheep possess some C activity. Thus, the serum of a bovine fetus only 12 cm in length was found to be slightly hemolytic, and this potency increased during gestation so that, at birth, serum titers were about one-fifth the level of adult cows. Studies by Colten and others with fetal sheep serum revealed detectable C1 activity on the 39th day of gestation, and here too the titers increased with age to attain adult C1

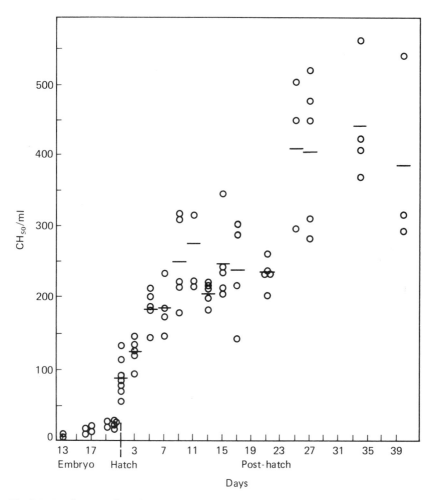

Fig. 5-1. Development of total complement activity in Line 96 chickens. CH_{50}/ml is plotted for each sample (an individual serum except for the early embryo pools of two or, rarely, three individual sera). Beginning on day 3 five animals were bled. (From A. E. Gabrielsen, R. J. Pickering, T. J. Linna, and R. A. Good, *Immunology* **25**:181, 1973.)

levels within a few days postpartum. A similar progression has been observed in the human for C1 and total serum activity, as well as for Factor B in the sera of rats. The sera of 14-day-old fetuses are hemolytic, and titers of cord blood serum at birth are about half of adult levels. Hemolytic activity for C1, C4, and C2 has been demonstrated in the sera of 8-week-old fetuses. C3 activity was demonstrable after 14 weeks.

These studies seem to indicate that there is little if any maternal transmission of hemolytic C activity, but more extensive analyses, particularly of the individual components, are required to further our understanding of the ontogeny of C in warm-blooded animals.

Several laboratories have linked the synthesis of C components to the H-2 gene in mice and the HL-A system in humans. Further studies of this important association should provide significant clues as to the possibility that some of the C components serve a critical recognition function similar to that of antigen receptors on bone marrow-derived lymphocytes.

Attempts to identify the sites of C synthesis in fetal and adult tissues have also been productive. As indicated by Rapp and Borsos, theoretically valid data in this area should meet several criteria. These include correlative hemolytic and immunochemical analyses, the use of functionally purified components in an appropriately designed assay, demonstration of specific incorporation of radio-labeled amino acids into the biologically active molecules, treatment of tissue to reduce preformed base-line levels, studies of the effects of metabolic inhibitors, and the accumulation of data which clearly distinguish between release and synthesis of the components in tissue cultures. These criteria have not always been fulfilled. The following section summarizes present findings, taken largely from the work of Colten and co-workers.

C1

When human and guinea pig intestinal tissues are preincubated with EDTA, preformed C1 levels are reduced to less than one molecule per tissue culture cell. Under these conditions, it was possible to demonstrate a thousandfold increment of C1 through application of a modified hemolytic plaque assay. These assays also helped localize the sites of C1 synthesis to the columnar epithelial cells of the small intestine, ileum, and colon as observed in 19-week-old fetal tissue. Since C1 is assembled through the interaction of C1q, C1r, and C1s, the possibility must be entertained that these subunits may represent products of different cells. Indeed, Laurell and her co-workers reported that $C\overline{1s}$ was synthesized in cultures of Hela cells and human fibroblasts in the absence of detectable amounts of C1q. This qualification gains further currency from reports of specific deficiencies in C1q and C1r, the former in a patient with lymphopenic agammaglobulinemia. A C1r deficit was observed in another individual, but in both patients the remaining C1 subunits were at normal levels. Kohler has reported that C1q synthesis was almost exclusively limited to fetal spleen cell cultures. Synthesis was detected by autoradiographic techniques based on the incorporation of [^{14}C] lysine and isoleucine and detection of the component with a monospecific antiserum in immunoelectrophoretic analyses. Synthesis of C1q began later in gestation than did C3, C4, or C5. In adults, C1 synthesis was not limited to the spleen since a decreased level of this component, relative to that of C3, C4, and C5, did not occur after splenectomy.

C4 *and* C2

The C2 component is apparently produced by a variety of cells. Synthesis of C2 has been found in cultured fragments of spleen and lungs, as well as in macrophages and cells from peritoneal exudates and bone marrow. The complexity of the problem in terms of cell identification is illustrated by the observation that peritoneal cells obtained by washing or from exudates induced by starch are far more productive of C2 than cells from oil- or casein-induced exudates. These findings may be taken to indicate heterogeneity among macrophages and do not exclude these cells in C2 biosynthesis. Ilgen and Burkholder isolated C4-synthesizing cells from guinea pig liver, spleen, and lungs. The C4-synthesizing cells were characterized as macrophages and were distinguished from antibody-producing cells in terms of their buoyant densities.

Mononuclear cells from peritoneal exudates also synthesize C4, the rate approximating 50×10^8 molecules per 10^6 cells per day. A valuable approach to questions of C component biosynthesis has been initiated by Colten and Parkman. Hybrid cells obtained by fusion of two cell lines, each of which was incapable of C4 synthesis, produced hemolytically active and immunochemically identifiable C4. The parent cells were furnished by peritoneal exudates from C4-deficient guinea pigs and a cell line of human origin, HeLa. The guinea pig cells synthesized C2 but not C4 in tissue culture. The human-guinea pig hybrid cells were characterized in terms of karyotype, presence of guinea pig membrane antigens, and susceptibility to lysis by C and antibody to guinea pig serum proteins. The biosynthesis of C4 as well as of C2 was inhibited by chemical carcinogens like 4-nitroquinoline-n-oxide, but not by their noncarcinogenic analogues.

C3

Direct evidence for synthesis of C3 in fetal tissues has been provided by Propp and Alper. They studied the concentration of paired maternal and cord sera for C3 and C3 allotypes by immunoelectrophoretic procedures with monospecific antisera. In twenty-five such pairs, the allotype of seven cord sera differed from that in the mother. In confirmation of other reports, the concentration of C3 in the cord sera was about half of that in the maternal sera, again suggestive of C3 synthesis by fetal tissues. In Kohler's experience, C3 synthesis was detectable in the 11-week-old fetus.

Adult liver tissues apparently synthesize C3 as judged by changes in C3 allotype following orthotopic human liver transplants. C3 synthesis has also been observed in a variety of human lymphoid tissues.

C5

Fetal synthesis of C5 was detected by Kohler in some instances after eight weeks of gestation and more regularly thereafter. The data in Fig. 5-2 taken from this report describe the ontogenesis of C1q, C3, C4, and C5 and of the IgG and IM immunoglobulins. Of interest is the finding that the biosynthesis of these C components precedes the appearance of immunoglobulins in human sera. Since the C system can be activated in the apparent absence of antibody, as shown in Chapter 3, these data support the conclusion that the C system provides a more primitive host defense system than that derived from antibody. Mice from a strain congenitally deficient in C5 synthesized this component for a short time following bone marrow transplants from allogeneic or coisogeneic donors.

Marked differences have been observed in the hemolytic C titers of male and female mice, as shown in Table 5-1. The sera of adult female mice of four inbred strains showed lower C titers than their age-controlled males. The diminution in the overall hemolytic activities has been attributed to differences in levels of C5 and C6. Hormonal control of the

Table 5–1

Complement and component titers in sera of inbred mice *

Strain	Sex †	CH_{50} per ml	$C\bar{I}H_{50}$ per ml $\times 10^5$	C3 ‡ percent hemolysis
Balb/c AnN	M	5.5	4.5	48.0
	F	2.5	3.5	4.1
C57BL/10ScN	M	3.3	2.4	65.6
	F	0.52	3.1	5.2
B10 D2/Sn "new"	M	>5.0	2.2	56.2
	F	0.47	2.8	9.4
B10 D2/Sn "old"	M	<0.2	2.7	0.0
	F	<0.1	3.3	0.0
DBA/2JN	M	<0.2	3.0	3.6
	F	<0.2	1.9	1.0
C57BL/6JN	M	1.3	2.7	29.6

* From W. D. Terry, T. Borsos, and H. J. Rapp, *J. Immunol.*, **92**:576, 1964.
† Adult mice, age range 3 to 8 months.
‡ Older terminology referring to components C3 through C9.

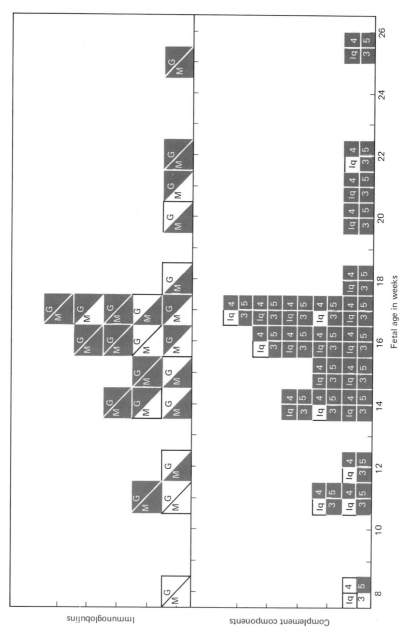

Fig. 5-2. Composite summary of protein synthesis by the individual fetuses. Blackened squares indicate synthesis of the complement protein (below) and blackened triangles synthesis of IgG and/or IGM (above). While synthesis of C3, C4, and C5 was uniformly present from 11 wk gestation onward, immunoglobulin synthesis was inconstant and quantitatively much less. In three fetuses, ages 8, 11, and 16 wk, complement but not IgG or IgM synthesis occurred. From P. Kohler, J. Clin. Invest. **52:**676, 1973.)

synthesis of these components has been invoked to explain the data of Table 5-1 since the sera of castrated or estrogen-treated male mice possess about the same activity as females. Conversely, the activity of sera from female mouse is increased after treatment with testosterone. Similar sex-related differences in C activity have been reported by Cinader and his colleagues who found that the serum titers of male Balb/cJ strain mice exceeded those of the females even at six weeks of age. The hybrid-cell technique introduced by Colten has been applied experimentally in a demonstration of "genetic repair." Macrophages from the spleens of C5-deficient mice and kidney cells from normal mice were used to generate hybrid cells. These cells elaborated C5 *in vitro* and restored the hemolytic C5 function in mice lacking this component.

The data in Table 5-1 have been considerably extended by the studies of Démant and others which led these investigators to conclude that the Ss-Slp region of the mouse genome is involved in the expression of hemolytic C activity. Their data, shown in Table 5-2, indicate that mice with the Ss^h-Slp^a allele have the highest C levels and that C titers are not correlated with the H-2K, H-2D, or Ir genotypes.

Table 5–2

Relative complement levels in males of H-2 congenic mouse strains *

Strain	H-2 haplo-type	Genotype				Recom-binant be-tween †	Number tested	Complement	
		H-2K	Ir-1	Ss-Slp	H-2D			level	±SE ‡
B10.A	a	k	k	h-a	d	k/d	22	1.67	±0.12 §
B10.D2/n	d	d	d	h-a	d	—	23	1.80	±0.13 §
B10.D2(R103)	g	d	d	h-a	b	d/b	5	2.25	±0.31 §
B10.A(2R)	h-2Sg	k	k	h-a	b	a/b	27	2.21	±0.22 §
B10.A(5R)	i	b	b	h-a	d	b/a	20	2.66	±0.34 §
C57BL/10Sn	b	b	b	h-o	b	—	49	1.00	±0.05
B10.A(4R)	h-3Sg	k	k	h-o	b	a/b	3	1.02	±0.10
B10.M	f	f	f	h-o	f	—	9	0.74	±0.13
B10.BR	k	k	k	l-o	k	—	23	0.61	±0.08 §
B10.AKM	m	k	k	l-o	q	k/q	10	0.64	±0.11 §
B10.HTT	tl	s	k	l-o	d	s/al	8	0.25	±0.03 §
C3H.OH	oh	d	d	h-a	k	d/k	3	1.75	±0.19 §
C3H.OL	ol	d	d	l-o	k	d/k	3	0.41	±0.14 ‖

* From P. Démant, J. Capková, E. Hinzová, and B. Vorácová, *Proc. Nat'l. Acad. Sci. U.S.A.*, **70**:863, 1973.

† When a strain carries a recombinant H-2 haplotype, the two original H-2 haplotypes between which the crossing-over occurred are given.

‡ Complement level relative to the C57BL/10Sn strain. The average complement level in C57BL/10Sn strain was 53.1 CH_{50} units at hemolysin dilution 1:200.

§ Significantly ($P \leq 0.01$, *t*-test) different from C57BL/10Sn.

‖ Significantly ($P \leq 0.01$, *t*-test) different from C3H.OH.

C6 *and* C9

Synthesis of these components by a rat hepatoma cell line has been reported. The evidence for C9 is more definitive in terms of characterization of the product and in the demonstration of a differential effect of hydrocortisone on the cultured cells. This steroid stimulated the synthesis of albumin but not of C9.

A recent report by Colten and collaborators indicated that cultures of four different rat hepatoma cells synthesized C2, C3, C5, and $\overline{\text{C1}}$INH.

PHYLOGENY OF THE C SYSTEM

In Invertebrates

Dr. Day and associates have reported that the hemolymph of invertebrates can be activated by the same constituent in cobra venom which initiates lysis of unsensitized erythrocytes via the C3 Activator ($\overline{\text{B}}$) system. Although hemolytic activity through the classical pathway is lacking, it is of interest from an evolutionary viewpoint that the hemolymphs of the horseshoe crab and sipunculid worm can be activated by cobra venom for the lysis of unsensitized erythrocytes. As with mammalian sera, the cobra venom factor was shown to form a complex with these hemolymphs which lysed sheep erythrocytes in the presence of EDTA-frog serum. The reaction resembles the mammalian system in that complex formation was inhibited by EDTA while the lytic reaction was suppressed in the presence of salicyladoxime.

In Vertebrates

Data pertaining to the activities of both the classical and alternate pathways for several species (vertebrates and invertebrates) are given in Table 5-3. While important facets of the C pathways in the various species remain to be elucidated, it is clear that both routes of C activation have a long evolutionary history. The presence of the alternate pathway in the invertebrate hemolymph points to the existence of host defense mechanisms prior to the appearance of specific immunoglobulins.

Phylogenetic studies of the C1 esterase inhibitor have been carried out by Drs. Virginia Donaldson and Jack Pensky. The functional properties attributed to the inhibitor (an α-2 neuramino glycoprotein) were detectable in plasma or serum from the fish, turtle, fowl, and several nonprimate as well as primate animals. The structures of these inhibitory substances

Table 5-3

Complement related lytic activity in sera of various species *

Category	Species studied	CH$_{50}$ per ml †	CoFH ‡ per ml	Natural lysins § for erythrocytes of:	Temperature dependency, °C	Potentiation by antibody	Heat stability	Cobra venom activation Lysis	Cobra venom activation C consumed
Vertebrates Mammalia	Guinea pig	1500–2000	40–80	Variety of mammalia	30–37	Usually by rabbit, g. pig, dog, cat	Labile 56°C	Yes	Yes
Aves	Chicken	52–90	110–160						
Reptilia	Cobra Turtle	150–200 2000–3000	<5 <5	Sheep, human	15–37	Rabbit and snake	Labile 6 min at 56°C	No	Yes
Amphibia	Frog	300–500	1000–1500	Goldfish, turtle, duck, rabbit, sheep, dog, human	4–28	Rabbit and turtle	Labile 20 min at 48°C	Yes	Yes
Osteichthyes	Carp Paddlefish	100–150 50–75	<5 <5	Goldfish, turtle, rabbit, sheep, dog	4–28	Variable	Labile 15 min at 53°C	No	No
Chondrichthyes	Nurse shark	300–400	<5	Goldfish, turtle, chicken, rabbit, sheep	25–30	Shark and turtle	Labile 20 min at 48°C	No	Yes
Agnatha	Lamprey Hagfish	<2 <2	<5 20–40	Sheep and rabbit	4	No	Stable 2.5 hr at 53°C	Yes	
Invertebrates Arthropoda	Horseshoe crab	<2	12–24						
Echinodermata	Starfish		>5						
Annelida	Sipunculid worm	<2	2.5–5.0						

* Modified from I. Gigli and K. F. Austen, Ann. Rev. Microbiol., **25**:309, 1971, and N. K. B. Day et al., J. Exp. Med., **132**:941, 1970.

† Classical immune hemolysis.

‡ Cobra venom inducible hemolysis.

§ Not restored with calcium, magnesium.

evidently differed among the several species since immunological identity was observed among the $\overline{C1}$ inhibitors of the human chimpanzee and gibbon but not with those of the baboon and rhesus monkeys. The squirrel monkey inhibitor seems to lack one or more antigens of the human protein, while the inhibitor in the plasmas of the lower species apparently had no immunologic relationship to the human preparation.

Studies with sera of apes and humans showed no antigenic differences in the components C1s, C4, C2, C3, C5, C6, C8, C9, and properdin Factor B. The components C1q, C1s, C4, C3, C8, and C9 in old-world monkeys, however, differed antigenically and in varying degrees from those in human sera. The sera of Prosimians differed in all components. Since hemolytic studies did not parallel the immunochemical findings, a dissociation between functional and antigenic sites was postulated by Schur and co-workers.

METABOLISM OF C COMPONENTS

The C proteins comprise slightly less than 10% by weight of human and guinea pig plasma proteins and it is reasonable to assume that their serum concentrations reflect an equilibrium between synthesis, release, and breakdown as do other plasma constituents. Human studies with isotopically labeled C1q, C3, C4, and C5 show fractional catabolic rates ranging from about 1 to 3% per hour of the total plasma pool. These values which represent a turnover of about 50% of the intravascular levels per day are slightly greater than those observed for other plasma proteins. Perhaps they reflect the continued consumption of C by the myriad number of antigen-antibody systems operating at low levels in the normal host economy. If this interpretation is correct, further studies of the role of C in tissue alteration and repair may provide a fruitful research area. This inference is strengthened by the demonstration that the rates of C3 and C4 synthesis, calculated to be in the range of 0.45 to 2.7 mg per kilogram per hour, are significantly lower in patients with disorders involving *in vivo* C utilization, such as systemic lupus erythematosus (SLE), hereditary angioedema, and hypocomplementemic glomerulonephritis. Pertinent data along these lines are provided in a report by Kohler and Müller-Eberhard on the metabolism of human C1q. These investigators monitored the *in vivo* metabolism of radioiodinated C1q in healthy adults and in patients with hypogammaglobulinemia, multiple myeloma, and SLE. The metabolic behavior of ^{125}C1q in the latter group of patients differed from the normals in that a greater loss of radioactivity was observed. Evidence was also obtained for a reversible binding of C1q with the plasma proteins, pointing to a significant uptake of C1q into the C1q,r,s, complex. Further, the plasma levels of C1q in the normals were two to three times higher than in the patients with hypogammaglobulinemia and multiple myeloma, and this finding was in accord with the higher catabolic rates of C1q in the latter two disorders. The rates of C1q synthesis were also higher in the patients than in the controls. The lower level of C1q in SLE was attributed to its consumption by the multiple immune reactions characteristic of this disease. In hypogammaglobulinemia and multiple myeloma, however, the lower C1q levels were associated with elevated catabolic rates and increased vascular distribution. As in earlier studies, the metabolism of C1q seemed to be governed by serum IgG concentrations. In hypogammaglobulinemia, limited interaction of C1q with IgG at ratios of one-to-five or six occurs, thereby accounting for the rapid clearance of the isotopically labeled C1q from the intravascular compartment. The findings for C1q do not necessarily apply to C1s since studies by Stroud and others suggest that there are distinct modes of synthesis or, possibly, catabolism of these subunits. The lowered C1q levels still allowed for mediation of some C functions. These aspects of C functions are discussed in greater detail in later chapters.

The parameters for the metabolic behavior of guinea pig C3 have also been established by Atkinson and others. They reported that the fractional catabolic rate was $7.9 \pm 4\%$ per hour, while the synthetic rate was 6.21 ± 0.43 mg per kilogram per hour. The percentage of C3 in the intravascular pool was $51 \pm 2\%$. These values and the serum levels of C3 were similar in conventional and C4-deficient guinea pigs. Lower catabolic rates for human C3 and Factor B (1.66% and 1.98% of the plasma pool per hour) were reported by Charlesworth and collaborators, who also estimated the synthetic rates of these two C proteins as 0.81 and 0.18 mg per kilogram per hour.

Genetic Aspects

This area of C studies has attracted the attention of an increasing number of investigators in recent years and has been well summarized in a review by Alper and Rosen. The isolation and characterization of the individual components which comprise the classical and alternate C systems have set the stage for the present state of our understanding. When chemically purified components become available in the quantities needed for structural studies, information of considerable importance to our understanding of the genetics of the C system and its role in maintaining normal tissue functions will become attainable.

C1q *Deficiency*

No inherited deficiency of this C subunit has been reported but C1q levels are usually depressed in patients with X-linked agammaglobulinemia and are usually correlated with the hypogammaglobulinemic state. Patients with immunodeficiency due to congenital lymphopenia and X-linked hypo-gammaglobulinemia do have very low C1q levels, but the mechanism of this deficiency is not well understood. A lack of this subunit has also been reported in two cases of acquired agammaglobulinemia ascribable to hyper-catabolism rather than diminished synthetic rates.

C1r *Deficiency*

This deficiency, described by Stroud and co-workers, was found in two brothers and a sister. In one sibling, the absence of C1r was associated with glomerulonephritis. In the other, the renal disease was also accompanied by skin and joint symptoms. The latter symptoms were prominent in the sister, who also experienced recurrent ear and respiratory infections. Five other living siblings were in apparent good health. The sera of the three affected individuals lacked hemolytic, bactericidal and immune adherence activity due to virtual absence of C1r. C1q and C1s levels were about half of normal. Full serologic function was restored with C1r. As might be expected, the deficiency of C1r did not affect activation of the alternate pathway. Genetically, this disorder has been attributed to an autosomal recessive mode of transmission. The deficiency of this sub-component was reflected in the inability of the patients' sera to mediate immune hemolysis. Whereas the CH_{50} and $\overline{C1}H_{50}$ titers were estimated at 227 ± 43 and $187,500 \pm 116,600$ in other family members, the values for the two homozygotes with a C1r deficiency were zero and 5000 respectively.

Hereditary Angioedema

One of the best-studied disorders associated with a genetic deficiency of a C-component inhibitor, $\overline{C1}$INH, was first described by Donaldson and Evans. Many of the clinical and immunologic features associated with this deficiency have been studied by Austen and his collaborators. Individuals with this disorder experience sudden episodes of edema which may affect the gastrointestinal and respiratory tracts, often with life-threatening consequences. Donaldson and Evans showed that the disease (HAE) was transmitted by an autosomal dominant factor associated with the absence of the $C\bar{1}$ esterase inhibitor, $C\bar{1}$INH. The presence of this inhibitor is assayed in terms of its capacity to block the hydrolysis of N-acetyl tyrosine ethyl ester or N-α-acetyl-L-lysine methyl ester by the $C\bar{1}$ esterase. A hemolytic assay is also available based on the inhibition of EAC14 or EAC142 formation from its precursors. $C\bar{1}$INH serum levels may also be estimated immunochemically in quantitative gel diffusion assays with a specific antiserum. This method is useful in detecting genetic polymorphism, but it furnishes little information regarding the functional properties of $C\bar{1}$INH.

The concentration of $C\bar{1}$INH in normal subjects has been estimated at about 200 μg per ml of serum. In the affected individuals, the level may be less than 25 μg per ml. The sera of about 15% of affected patients or their kindred contain a biologically inactive form of $C\bar{1}$INH. The sera of some patients and their family members possess normal or even elevated levels of $C\bar{1}$INH in an altered state as judged by abnormal electrophoretic mobility due to noncovalent binding with serum albumin.

Edema production in patients with HAE is attributed to activation of the $C\bar{1}$ esterase in plasma and is associated with depletion of C4 and C2, particularly during the symptomatic period. The nature of the initiating stimulus for this activation has not been identified. C3 levels are usually within the normal range. Edema formation results from separation of the endothelial cells lining the postcapillary venules and can be reproduced by the intradermal injection of purified $C\bar{1}$ in both man and guinea pigs and in C2-deficient humans. Klemperer and others consider that the edema is due to a vasoactive peptide liberated as a result of the $C\bar{1}$, C4, and C2 interaction. Amino acid composition studies show that this peptide differs from bradykinin. This peptide also differs from bradykinin in its susceptibility to destruction by trypsin and inhibition of its formation by antisera to C4 or C2, but not to C3. The work of Donaldson and others implicates the fibrinolytic and kallikrein systems in the activation of C1 and in the generation of the agent implicated in hereditary angioedema.

In studies with purified Hageman factor and $C\bar{1}$INH, Donaldson established a relationship between this constituent of the blood clotting system and activation of $C\bar{1}$. In brief, activation of the clot-promoting factor induced formation of $C\bar{1}$ in the plasma of patients with HAE but not with that of normal individuals. Donaldson also implicated the kinin system in both blood coagulation and $C\bar{1}$ activation. The current thought is that activation of the Hageman factor by glass surfaces or ellagic acid triggers the clotting and kinin-forming systems. One product of these reactions involves the conversion of plasminogen into plasmin, an enzyme shown to convert C1 into its esterostatic form, $C\bar{1}$. The validity of this sequence is supported by the demonstration that epsilon amino caproic acid, an inhibitor of plasminogen activation to plasmin, is clinically useful in the treatment of HAE.

The interrelationships between the blood-clotting, kinin-generating, and C systems are discussed in Chapter 8.

C4 Deficiency

In man   Several authors have now recorded a deficiency of C4 in a few Swiss and Japanese individuals. This deficit was found in the sera of 14 of 41,083 young Swiss men and in 3 of 42,000 Japanese individuals. In the latter three cases, the deficiency was expressed in terms of hemolytic but not antigenic activity. Thus Torisu and his colleagues detected a line in the βIE region in immunoelectrophoretic assays with anti-C4, but the hemolytic activity in the sera of these individuals was diminished by more than 90%. Although the meaning of these findings is not clear, they may be related to studies in Austen's laboratory in which the existence of nine polymorphic variants of C4 has been postulated on the basis of immunoelectrophoretic assays. These experiments also strengthened the evidence for fetal synthesis of C4 since in five of nine paired maternal and cord sera, the C4 subtype of the newborn was absent in the mother. Rosenfeld and others have described ten patterns in the electrophoretic mobility of C4 whose significance in terms of heritable and quantitative features has not yet been evaluated.

In guinea pigs   In their search for allotypic antibodies, Ellman, Frank, and their colleagues found a male guinea pig whose serum apparently lacked C4, since the animal synthesized antibody to C4 following immunization with whole guinea pig serum. A screening of 250 guinea pigs with this antiserum revealed five additional animals deficient in this component. When the C4-deficient animals were bred with normal or other C4-deficient guinea pigs, it became apparent that the trait was transmitted as an autosomal recessive characteristic in which the heterozygous state was readily discernible. Evidence in support of these interpretations is supplied in Fig. 5-3.

The sera of C4-deficient animals lacked the ability to lyse sensitized sheep red cells due to the absence of hemolytically active C4. The plasma protein corresponding to this component was also missing. Neither was a nonfunctional antigenic variant of this protein detectable. The species specificity of C4 was also demonstrated by Frank and others, since the guinea pig antiserum to C4 failed to react with C4 preparations of rabbits, mice, cats, goats, or humans (with one exception). In heterozygous guinea pigs, the hemolytic C4 levels ranged from 8 to 30% of the normal values.

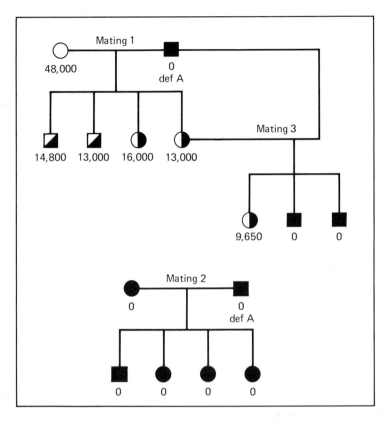

Fig. 5-3. Results of matings of C4-deficient guinea pigs with normal, C-4-deficient, or heterozygous-deficient guinea pigs. The C4 titer is shown below each symbol; ○ = normal, ◑ = heterozygous-deficient, ● = homozygous-deficient animals. (From M. M. Frank et al., *5th Int'l. Symposium Canadian Society for Immunology,* Guelph, 1970, S. Karger, Basel, 1972, p. 256.)

Further studies of the C4-deficient guinea pigs provided a considerable body of interesting data. Thus, the reaction systems involving allergic responses of both the immediate (passive cutaneous anaphylactic and Arthus reactions) and of the delayed (tuberculin and contact sensitivity) types were not weakened in these animals. In contrast, clearance of ^{51}Cr-labeled autologous or isologous erythrocytes sensitized with rabbit antiserum was considerably delayed. Early antibody production to bovine serum albumin but not to other antigens seems to have been impaired in the C4-deficient guinea pigs. Since these assays were carried out by the Farr technique, this finding may only reflect differences in antibody avidity. Significantly, later antibody synthesis was not depressed. Nor was the antibody-forming capacity to dinitrophenylated bovine gamma globulin diminished as judged by quantitative precipitin assays. It would seem, then, that a deficiency in C4 does not weaken the humoral and cellular defense mechanisms of these guinea pigs, a conclusion consonant with their general state of health and viability.

The availability of the C4-deficient guinea pigs provided an unusual opportunity to confirm the earlier reports as to the existence of the alternate or properdin C pathways. Thus, component utilization in endotoxin-treated, homozygous C4-deficient serum was confined to the late-acting components, C5 to C9. With serum from heterozygotes, some consumption of C1 and C4 was observed. The findings with immune complexes were of interest since the fixation of C1 and C2 proceeded to the same extent with sera of normal guinea pigs or those with a heterozygous or homozygous deficiency. Since the homozygous deficiency is characterized by the complete absence of C4, fixation of C1 and C2 can be rationalized as follows. The immune complexes convert C1 to $\overline{C1}$ and this enzyme, as stated earlier, can cleave C2 in the fluid phase. However there is no formation of the $\overline{C42}$ convertase; so the consumption of the later components must be attributed to the activity of the C3 proactivator or properdin pathway. The validity of this interpretation can be established by immunologic depletion of C1 and C2 in the C4-deficient sera. The need for experiments of this type is indicated by the observation that the C4-deficient sera supported the immune adherence reaction, which is known to depend on formation of the intermediate C423b.

In rats Arroyave and his colleagues have recently reported a C4-deficit in the sera of some male Wistar rats. These sera contained 20% or less of the activity detectable in other animals of the same strain. Addition of purified human C4 fully restored the hemolytic activity. The C4 deficiency was found in ten of thirty males, but in none of twenty females screened for this characteristic. An autosomal recessive mode of transmission has been postulated with a gene dosage effect.

C2 *Deficiency in Man*

Five human kindreds whose sera are deficient in C2 have been reported. For a time these findings were of interest because the specific deficiency was not associated with any clinical manifestations, a seemingly anomalous situation in view of the role of C in host defense. The discovery of alternate C pathways erased this paradox. The deficiency, studied by Klemperer, is due to the lack of hemolytically active C2 and not to the presence of an inhibitor. The sera of homozygous individuals are hemolytically inert due to the lack of the C2 protein as judged by several methods, including its detection with monospecific antiserum. Serum levels of 1 to 4% have, however, been reported in some homozygotes, in experiments based on the uptake of isotopically labeled components. In the heterozygotes, serum C2 levels range from about 30 to 60% of the normal values. Immunologic reactions, such as immune adherence, which require C2 may be depressed in the sera of homozygotic individuals, yet some of them now in the sixth decade of life show no unusual susceptibility to infection.

A study of C2 protein concentration as a function of hemolytic site formation by Ruddy and others led to the interesting finding that 1 μg of this component could form as many as 4×10^{10} effective C2 sites. Assuming chemical homogeneity, it was calculated that 130 molecules of C2 are required to produce one hemolytically active site. It would follow that the sera of individuals with a homozygous deficiency possess fewer molecules of C2 than these threshold values. In conformity with studies of other components, cord blood assays failed to reveal any maternal transmission of this component.

C3 Deficiency

In guinea pigs   In 1919 Moore found a strain of guinea pigs whose sera lacked hemolytic activity (ca. 1% of normal levels). Follow-up studies by Hyde and others suggested that this deficiency was due to the component then called C'3, since zymosan-treated normal guinea pig serum failed to restore hemolytic activity. In the light of present knowledge, the specificity of this deficit cannot be accurately defined. The deficiency was inherited as a simple Mendelian recessive trait, a pioneering discovery in the inheritance of a non-sex-linked factor in mammalian serum. Despite a reduction in the opsonic activity of the serum, the deficient animals generally fared as well as the controls. Unfortunately, a naturally occurring streptococcal infection almost wiped out the entire laboratory colony; consequently, definitive studies regarding the nature of this deficiency could not be pursued as refinements in C technology became available. A few salient facts did emerge. There was no placental transmission of the deficiency. Moreover, the affected guinea pigs showed the same susceptibility as did the normals to anaphylactic reactions but not to Forssman shock induced by the intravenous or subcutaneous injections of rabbit antiserum to chicken red cells.

In man: Genetic polymorphism   Electrophoretic analyses of fresh human sera by Wieme in 1965 suggested that C3 activity might be associated with proteins of different mobilities. At about the same time,

Ropartz and others reported that a small percentage of human sera agglutinated tanned red cells coated with C3. Since the sera of other individuals inhibited this agglutination, a genetic polymorphism of this component was suggested, although these findings were not accompanied by family studies. Alper and Propp investigated these phenomena more extensively and they with others have uncovered the existence of at least eighteen forms of C3 differing in their electrophoretic mobilities in agarose gels. Initially they found two variants called C3S (slow) and C3F (fast), the former being most common. Some uncertainty was temporarily introduced due to the binding of calcium by C3. This difficulty has since been resolved and eighteen variants have now been described in terms of their relative electrophoretic mobilities as shown in Fig. 5-4. Gene frequency studies indicate that C3F is a Caucasian gene since it occurs but rarely in Oriental populations, as shown in Table 5-4.

All of the variants studied thus far appear to function normally, a finding consistent with the observation that the polymorphism is associated with the largest conversion product of C3. One of the minor fragments, C3a, associated with anaphylatoxic activity has the same electrophoretic mobility whether prepared from C3F or C3S. C3 polymorphism has also been detected in a limited number of sera from the monkey, *Macaca mulatta,* and like their human counterparts, the genes are inherited as autosomal codominant traits.

Genetic studies are available for three generations of one kindred in whom seven of twenty-two individuals had approximately half-normal levels of C3. These individuals show no unusual susceptibility to infection.

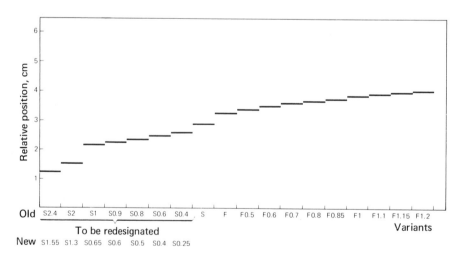

Fig. 5-4. C3 variants as detected in prolonged agarose gel electrophoresis. ("Statement on the Polymorphism of the Third Component of Complement in Man," *Vox Sang.* **25:**18, 1973.)

Table 5–4

C3 gene frequencies *

Population	No. sera examined	S	F
North American			
Caucasian	472	0.77	0.22 or 0.21
Norwegian	400	0.80	0.19
German	226	0.78	0.19
North American			
Negro	154	0.92–0.96	0.07–0.04
North American			
Oriental	68	0.99	—

* From C. A. Alper and F. S. Rosen, *Advances in Immunology,* 14:251, 1971.

The analyses of Alper and Rosen show that serum C3 levels are governed by two codominant genes, each of which is responsible for the synthesis of half the serum concentration. One patient has been identified with a homozygous deficiency who had undetectable serum levels of C3. The absence of this component was associated with an extreme susceptibility to bacterial infections which required twenty hospital admissions. The review by Alper and Rosen should be consulted for a more detailed statement.

C5 *Deficiency*

In mice   This deficiency was first described by Rosenberg and Tachibana in studies of several inbred strains. The genetic mechanism was shown to be controlled at a single locus in which the positive allele, Hc′, was dominant. Deficient mice were therefore homozygous. As was later shown for the C4-deficient guinea pigs, the C5-deficient mice, on immunization with normal mouse serum, produced antibodies which reacted specifically with a beta globulin in the immunizing serum. Cinader and Dubiski, in independent studies of allotypic serum proteins, described an antigen which they called MμB1. They found that the presence or absence of MμB1 could be correlated with the hemolytic activity of different mouse sera. Further experiments revealed identical physicochemical properties of Hc′ and MμB1. Both were heat-labile euglobulins, resistant to ammonia, hydrazine, 2-mercaptoethanol, and EDTA. The identity of these products with C5 was subsequently established by Nilsson and Müller-Eberhard who showed that mouse anti-MμB1 reacted with human C5. Further, an antiserum prepared in mice lacking MμB1 reacted only with the sera of mice which were hemolytically active and contained this antigen. Finally, the antisera to MμB1 and C5 gave reactions of identity in double-diffusion assays with human C5 and normal mouse serum. Later genetic analyses showed that the heterozygous C5-deficient mice had just about half of the serum concentration of C5 in age- and sex-matched homozygotic, normal mice.

Several inbred strains of mice lacking C5 have been available for studies of the role of C in blood clearance, graft rejection, opsonic activity, etc. Strangely, the lack of C5 did not seem to be associated with profound differences in the operations of the host defense apparatus. The coisogenic strain B10.D2/SN "old" line is C5-deficient, while the B10.D2/SN "new" line has normal levels of C5. A C5 deficient BALB/c strain is also available for studies of this type. An extensive set of data regarding the occurrence of the MμB1 antigen in various inbred mouse strains and its taxonomic distribution in mammals has been supplied by Cinader and his colleagues.

In man Miller and Nilsson studied two unrelated infants with a syndrome of eczematoid dermatitis, intractable diarrhea, recurrent infections due to gram-negative bacteria and staphylococcal sepsis. The sera of these infants failed to opsonize yeast particles, a defect restored by normal human serum and purified human C5 but not by C5-deficient mouse serum. The hemolytic and immunochemical characteristics of the patients' C5 were normal except, as mentioned, for the depressed phagocytosis. It has been suggested that this discrete dysfunction might be due to a depression of chemotactic activity by an altered 5a anaphylatoxin. Adult relatives of the propositi were healthy, and the mode of transmission of this genetic defect has not been established.

C6 *Deficiency*

In rabbits A heritable defect of this component in rabbits has been found in Germany (Rother and Rother, 1961), in Mexico (Biro and Ortega, 1966), and in England (Lachmann, 1970). The sera of the affected animals were neither anticomplementary nor inhibitory for the activity of normal rabbit serum, and the deficiency could be restored with purified C6. The C6 deficient sera contained the C6 inactivator, but not the C6 protein; so the deficient animals could synthesize specific antibodies for this component when immunized with normal rabbit serum. Lachmann's studies indicate that this deficiency is inherited as a single autosomal recessive trait. A deficiency in C6 has also been described by Yang and co-workers in individual strains of Golden Syrian hamsters.

In man   Leddy and collaborators reported the absence of C6 in a young female whose serum lacked the hemolytic as well as the antigenic properties of this component. The sera of the girl's parents and five of her six siblings had about half of the normal functional levels of C6. The absence of this component was associated with a complete lack of bactericidal activity for *Salmonella typhi* 0901 and *Hemophilus influenzae,* type b, and an inability to induce lysis of red cells from patients with paroxysmal nocturnal hemoglobinuria. Other functions such as generation of chemotactic activity and mediation of immune adherence were present and at normal levels.

ALTERNATE PATHWAY DYSFUNCTION

Only two abnormalities of the properdin system have thus far been described, both by Alper and his associates. The first concerns polymorphism in the glycine-rich β-glycoprotein (Factor B), which is considered as a four-allele autosomal codominant system. The genes, based on their electrophoretic mobilities, have been designated Gb^S, Gb^F, Gb^{S1}, and Gb^{F1}. The Gb^{S1} gene has been found only in Caucasians, and the Gb^{F1} gene, in Negroes.

A deficiency in one of the alternate pathway components was discovered in studies of a young man with recurrent pyogenic infections since infancy and Klinefelters's syndrome. C studies indicated a number of abnormalities associated with the C3 system whose underlying cause was eventually attributed to a genetic deficiency of the C3 inactivator in the following manner. The patient's serum possessed about 50% of the normal hemolytic C potency, i.e., 15 CH_{50}/ml, but lacked bactericidal and phagocytosis-enhancing activity. C-component assays indicated normal levels for all save C3 which was low, 280 μg/ml. Most of the C3 in the serum was in the form of C3b, the inactive cleavage product. Attempts to restore C-mediated functions to his serum by adding C3 were unsuccessful.

The rate of C3 synthesis by the patient was normal, but its catabolism was five times faster than normal and was attributed to a rapid *in vivo* cleavage. Further studies revealed that Factor B or C3PA was rapidly cleaved *in vitro,* being complete in ten minutes at 37° C. The fragmentation required magnesium. One of the *in vivo* abnormalities resulting from this process was the coating of the patient's cells with C3b, thereby enhancing their rate of clearance. An infusion of plasma restored the capacity of the patient's serum to mediate bactericidal and hemolytic reactions, promote phagocytosis and chemotaxis, and the patient's red cells lost their agglutinability with an anti-C3 serum. It is thus apparent that the patient's serum had several abnormalities: low C3, high C3 catabolic rate, low C3PA (properdin Factor B). These deficiencies were associated with the absence of the C3b inactivator, KAF, but additional abnormalities have not been excluded. This genetic abnormality has been called a type-I essential hypercatabolism of C3 to distinguish it from a rather similar situation, called Type II, which involves an enzyme that degrades C3.

FURTHER READING

Alper, C. A., and Rosen, F. S., "Genetic Aspects of the Complement System," *Advances in Immunology,* **14**:251, 1971.

Ballow, M., Fang, F., Good, R. A., and Day, N. K., "Developmental Aspects of Complement Components in the Newborn," *Clin. Exp. Immunol.* **18**:257, 1974.

Charlesworth, J. A., Williams, D. G., Sherington, E., Lachmann, P. J., and Peters, D. K., "Metabolic Studies of the Third Component of Complement and the Glycine-Rich Beta Glycoprotein in Patients with Hypocomplementemia, *J. Clin. Invest.,* **53**:1578, 1974.

Cinader, B., Dubiski, S., and Wardlaw, A. C., "Distribution of $M_\mu B1$ Antigen," *J. Exp. Med.,* **120**:897, 1964.

Day, N. K. B., Gewurz, H., Johansen, R., Finstad, J., and Good, R. A., "Complement Activity in Lower Vertebrates and Invertebrates," *J. Exp. Med.,* **132**:941, 1970.

Fat, R. F. M., Lai, A., and Van Furth, R, "In Vitro Synthesis of Some Complement Components (C1q, C3, and C4) by Lymphoid Tissues and Circulating Leucocytes in Man, *Immunology,* **28**:359, 1975.

First International Symposium and Workshop on the Polymorphism of the Third Component of the Human Complement System, *Vox. Sang.,* **25**:9, 1973.

Gigli, I., and Austen, K. F., "Phylogeny and Function of the Complement System," *Ann. Rev. Microbiol.,* **25**:309, 1971.

Ruddy, S., Gigli, I., and Austen, K. F., "The Complement System in Man," *New Eng. J. Med.,* **287**:489, 545, 592, and 642, 1972.

Stroud, R. M., "Genetic Abnormalities of the Complement System of Man Associated with Disease," *Transplantation Proc.,* **6**:59, 1974.

Chapter 6

Complement-mediated

Host Defense Mechanisms

This chapter deals with those functions of the C system concerned with host mechanisms of defense against invasive microorganisms. These include the direct attack on pathogenic agents through immune cytocidal reactions, phagocytosis, virus neutralization, as well as the possible role of C in the enhancement of antibody formation.

BACTERICIDAL REACTIONS

Unlike the immune hemolytic system, quantitative studies of the bactericidal action of C and antibody on gram-negative bacteria have encountered two major difficulties. Susceptible organisms such as the Escherichia, Salmonella, and Shigella genera possess an impervious cell wall which must be penetrated before the C attack mechanisms can be most effective. Secondly, these organisms multiply during the ongoing bacteriolytic process, thereby complicating a quantitative expression of the reaction. The simplest procedure for demonstrating bactericidal action involves incubation of a standardized cell suspension in the logarithmic growth phase with an excess of C and varying dilutions of the antiserum. The surviving bacteria are then enumerated by plating on agar or by optical measurements. Muschel and Treffers have used the latter method with S. *typhi* and recorded several similarities to immune hemolysis. These include a magnesium requirement, a reciprocal relationship between antibody and C, and the demonstration that only a few antibody molecules suffice to kill these organisms. One of the issues which troubled many students of this problem was the frequent failure to observe pronounced lysis of the bacteria despite their loss of viability, i.e., cell death was not equivalent to lysis. This issue was resolved by Amano, Inoue, and their associates, who irradiated the bacteria before subjecting them to immune bacteriolysis. The extent of lysis was then measured by estimating the release of nucleic acids into the supernates of reaction mixtures. Cell death due to C and antibody was accompanied by loss of phospholipids from the cells but not by lysis unless lysozyme was added to convert the rod-like bacteria into spheroplasts lacking cell walls. The spheroplasts were then transformed into ghosts by the lysozyme present in the sera or as a result of their inherent instability. Removal of lysozyme from the reaction mixtures by treatment of the antiserum and complement with bentonite permits the bactericidal effect to be observed in terms of colony counts, but bacteriolysis is not observed. Kinetic studies by Davis and others have demonstrated this succession of events which is illustrated in Fig. 6-1. This experiment was carried out with *E. coli* and human serum which probably provided both antibody and C. As may be seen, the number of viable organisms and rod-like forms decreased simultaneously and rapidly after an initial lag of about five minutes. The diminution in these parameters was not accompanied by marked changes in optical density. Coincidental with a drop in colony count and rod-like forms, a sharp increase in the number of spheroplasts was observed. The spheroplasts gave way, in turn, to bacterial ghosts. Under the conditions used in this experiment, a clear distinction was discerned between the bactericidal and bacteriolytic events. The incorporation of 0.005 M calcium chloride stabilized the spheroplasts with a marked delay in the appearance of the cell ghosts.

In later studies, Inoue and his collaborators demonstrated that all nine components of the C system are required for bacteriolysis. This finding was achieved through characterization of cell-bound C intermediates which were entirely analogous to those participating in immune hemolysis.

Bactericidal action can also proceed through activation of the properdin system as first demonstrated in Pillemer's studies, and confirmed in more recent studies which showed that bactericidal action can progress in C4-deficient guinea pig serum albeit at a slower rate than in conventional guinea pig serum. As discussed in Chapter 3, bacterial lipopolysaccharides are efficient initiators of the alternate pathway, but the killing of gram-negative bacteria by this route differs from the inability of the same activation sequence to lyse unsensitized erythrocytes. In all likelihood, the destruction of gram-negative bacteria, but not of the red cells, can be attributed to the presence of antibacterial immunoglobulins in the serum used as a C source. This is evident from the fact that the lipopolysaccharides utilize C1, C4, and C2 as well as the properdin pathway.

The complex structure of the cell walls of gram-negative bacteria has given rise to numerous studies designed to correlate the presence of surface antigens with pathogenicity and susceptibility to C-dependent bactericidal reactions. The findings of Glynn and Howard are of interest in this regard. They reported that the amount of K antigen (an acidic polysaccharide on the surface of many strains of *E. coli*) was inversely related

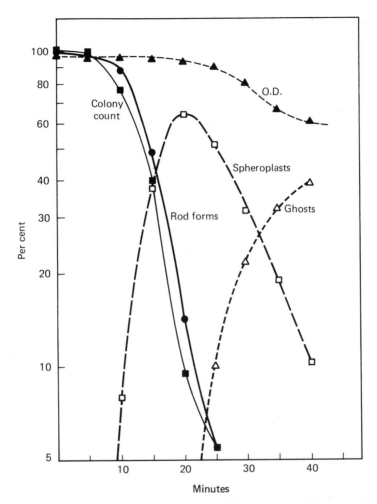

Fig. 6-1. Kinetics of changes in colony count, optical density, and transformation of bacterial rods to spheroplasts and ghosts. (From S. D. Davis, D. Gemsa, and R. J. Wedgwood, *J. Immunol.,* **96:**570, 1966.)

to the susceptibility of the organism to destruction by C and antibody. Of related interest is their observation that extracts of the K antigen inhibit the sensitization of erythrocytes by IgG or IgM hemolysins as well as lysis of the sensitized cells by C. It would appear that this membrane constituent acts by impeding the union of antibody to the red cell and, subsequently, the lytic action of the C system. Elucidation of the structural basis for these inhibitory properties should be of considerable interest.

The similarity in the mechanism of C action on erythrocytes and on gram-negative bacteria extends to the nature of the lesions produced in the two cell membranes. Characteristic lesions have been visualized on cells of *E. coli* and *V. alcalescens* following completion of the C sequence. The lesions produced with normal guinea pig serum resemble the holes formed in red cell membranes in their gross characteristics.

The development of the treponemal immobilization test by Nelson and Mayer provided unequivocal evidence of a role for serum antibody in immunity to syphilis. The immobilization of *Treponema pallidum* by C occurs after interaction with antibody has progressed for about 18 hours. Lysozyme accelerates this process presumably through digestion of a heavy polysaccharide layer which prevents rapid sensitization of the cell to action by C. An unequivocal example of the lysozyme effect was demonstrated by Metzger in experiments dealing with the immobilization of *Treponema pallidum* by antibody and C. In mixtures containing these reactants, 50% immobilization required a reaction time in excess of 18 hours at 37° C. The addition of 5 or 50 μg of egg-white lysozyme reduced the time needed for 50% immobilization to 8 and 5 hours, respectively. The similarity of these events to the mechanism described by Glynn for antigen K in *E. coli* is striking. A similar process occurs when leptospires are subjected to immune inactivation. Destruction of the integrity of the mucopeptide outer sheaths of these organisms by C and antibody permits lysozyme to attack the protoplasmic membrane and disrupt the cylindrical structure of these organisms.

PHAGOCYTOSIS

The discovery of this phenomenon by Metchnikoff was quickly followed by studies purporting to demonstrate the role of C in the ingestion of bacteria, particularly those of the gram-positive genera and others which resist immune bacteriolysis, and of antigen-antibody complexes by macrophages and polymorphonuclear cells. Much of the evidence, based on the use of fresh and heat-inactivated sera, indicated that the former accelerated and intensified the phagocytic process. The early experiments also showed that the serum factors which promote phagocytosis are largely due to specific antibody. Considerable effort has since been expended to suggest that phagocytosis plays a predominant role in combating infections such as pneumococcal pneumonia during the early or "pre-antibody" phase of the infection. In the light of present knowledge, activation of the alternate C pathway by the pneumococcal capsular polysaccharides can certainly be invoked as a possible mechanism. However, the difficulties that beset attempts to prove a null hypothesis are formidable since it is fairly well established that antibody synthesis is initiated within hours after antigenic stimulation, but detection of low levels of antibody during the early response requires highly sensitive and appropriate assay procedures. Moreover, the widespread cross-reactivities which characterize the polysaccharide immune systems provide another means of promoting *in vivo* phagocytosis from the very outset of the infectious process. The failure to inhibit opsonization by inclusion of an excess of the soluble type specific pneumococcal polysaccharide does not constitute rigorous evidence in this regard. Many investigators, working with a variety of immune systems, have been unable to deplete normal sera of their antibodies by repeated adsorptions with specific antigens. Support for these comments has recently been furnished by Winkelstein and Shin. They showed that the binding of guinea pig gamma-2 immunoglobulins to pneumococci was necessary to mediate the ingestion of these organisms by phagocytic cells presumably through activation of the alternate pathway by their $F(ab')_2$ fragments, as has been demonstrated in a number of other instances. These investigators also showed that C3 was fixed to the surface of the pneumococci and this event preceded opsonization. Activation of C3 was achieved through the properdin pathway. This process was considerably accelerated and intensified when the mediating IgG2 immunoglobulins were furnished by specifically immunized guinea pigs as compared to IgG2 derived from normal animals or from those immunized with a dinitrophenylated protein conjugate as illustrated in Fig. 6-2. In their experiments absorption of the guinea pig IgG2 preparations with type-25 pneumococci but not with *E. coli* diminished the phagocytic capacity of the antibody solution.

Identification of C's role in these events did not reach a decisive stage until Nelson clarified the mechanism of immune adherence. As discussed previously, and in later experiments with Gigli, Nelson showed that the binding of C3b to bacterial or other cell surfaces promoted their opsonization or ingestion by phagocytic cells. A graphic illustration was provided by Robineaux and Nelson, who visualized the *in vitro* phagocytosis of bacteria by human polymorphonuclear cells after the organisms had undergone immune adherence to human erythrocytes. These experiments strengthened the premise that immune adherence facilitates *in vivo* phagocytosis of microorganisms by cells from primates. Nonprimate platelets presumably serve the same function as primate erythrocytes in promoting phagocytosis through immune adherence.

Since the binding of C3b is essential for immune adherence, it was quite natural for investigators to look at the participation of the alternate pathway in phagocytosis. As has been suggested, the experiments of Winkelstein and others testify to the function of this C pathway. The results of a typical experiment are shown in Table 6-1 which is taken from

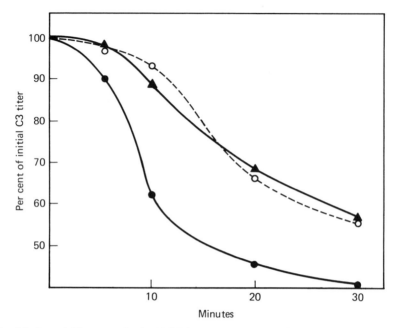

Fig. 6-2. Rate of C3 consumption in C4-deficient guinea pig serum by Type 25 pneumococci pretreated in buffer (O), normal (●), or immunospecific (▲), guinea pig serum. C4D GPS = C4-deficient guinea pig serum. (From J. A. Winkelstein and H. S. Shin, J. *Immunology* **112**: 1639, 1974.)

Table 6–1

Heat-Labile Opsonins to Type-25 Pneumococci in Normal and
C4-deficient Guinea Pig Serum *

Test medium	% Phagocytosis
Hanks' buffer—modified (HBG)	0
Normal guinea pig serum	
Undiluted	58
1:2 †	51
1:5	37
1:10	3
1:20	0
C4-deficient serum	
Undiluted	60
1:2 †	53
1:5	45
1:10	3
1:20	0

* J. A. Winkelstein, H. S. Shin, and W. B. Wood, Jr., J. *Immunol.*, **108**:1687, 1972.
† Diluted in HBG.

their report. These findings corroborate those reported by Shin and others in showing that depletion of C3 from normal mouse serum markedly depressed the heat-labile opsonic activity which could be restored by the incorporation of the purified component. The presence of C3 (or C3b) on the pneumoccocal surface was revealed by the quellung reaction with anti-C3. The presence of C5 was apparently of minor significance for *in vitro* phagocytosis, although C5-deficient mice were found to be materially more susceptible to infection by type-25 pneumococci.

The experimental results cited above based on the use of C4-deficient guinea pig serum agree with those performed by Root and others published at about the same time. These authors also found that sera lacking C4 promoted ingestion of *S. aureus,* Type-25 pneumococci, *E. coli,* and *C. albicans,* but at slower rates than those achieved with sera of normal animals or of those from guinea pigs which were heterozygous with respect to the C4 deficiency. Activation of the alternate C pathway was therefore considered sufficient to mediate this defense mechanism. The *in vitro* studies were supplemented by experiments which demonstrated that both normal and C4-deficient guinea pigs resisted challenge with large numbers of the pneumococci and *E. coli.* Since C5 also facilitates phagocytosis of pneumococci and yeast cells and since this reaction proceeds in C4-deficient animals, it seems that the later C components may participate through activation of the alternate pathway in such a manner that the components C3b and C5b are fixed to the microorganisms by a mechanism other than that requiring C1, C4, C2, and immune adherence. These considerations are supported by Jason, in whose hands opsonization of *E. coli* by heated serum was elevated by the incorporation of purified C3 proactivator. Forsgren and Quie implicated the alternate pathway in the phagocytosis of *S. aureus, E. coli,* and *C. albicans* on the basis of their observations that opsonic activity progressed in the presence of EGTA. Diamond and his colleagues compared the roles of the classical and alternate pathways in the phagocytosis of *Cryptococcus neoformans* by human leukocytes. They concluded that the classical mode of C activation accelerated the uptake of these organisms through the involvement of antibody and the early-acting components, C1, C4, and C2. However, the extent of phagocytosis was the same with both C-activation pathways.

The alternate pathway has also been implicated in the extraneural phagocytosis of cryptococci in guinea pigs by Diamond and his colleagues. Treatment of the animals with the cobra venom factor heightened the intensity of the infection as monitored by the number of fungi in the peripheral blood, lung, and liver. The late C components participated in the clearance of the organisms from these sites, but not from the brain tissues once the cryptococci gained access.

Erythrocytes containing C5 and C6 are also subject to phagocytosis in reactions involving IgA, IgG, and IgM as reported by Dalmasso, Frank, and their associates. IgG and IgM differ in their modes of action under *in vivo* conditions. Radiolabeled guinea pig erythrocytes sensitized with these hemolysins were sequestered in the liver and cleared from the blood at an accelerated rate when the cells contained a minimum of 60 C-fixing sites per cell as judged by $C\overline{1}$ fixation assays. The IgG hemolysins were more effective than their IgM counterparts in these experiments. As few as 1.4 C-fixing sites per cell sufficed to enhance blood clearance, with most of the sequestration occurring in the spleen. In C4-deficient guinea pigs, accelerated blood clearance was not observed with IgM and was greatly impaired with IgG antibodies. Depletion of the late-acting components in guinea pigs treated with cobra venom also decreased the rate of blood clearance. It was concluded that neither the classic nor the alternate pathway contributed to the accelerated clearance. Earlier evidence was cited to the effect that erythrocytes coated with C components are more resistant to lysis and may have normal survival times. These interpretational difficulties, stemming from *in vivo* studies, suggest the need for detailed analyses of the number and nature of the cell-bound C components as parameters governing the *in vivo* blood clearance.

M. Rabinovitch and his colleagues have pinpointed the role of C in phagocytosis by macrophages. Using ^{51}Cr-labeled sheep erythrocytes sensitized with rabbit antibody and mouse peritoneal macrophages, they showed that the antibody and C served separate functions. Addition of mouse serum to EA promoted attachment of the red cells to the macrophages, a process which was inhibited by anti-C3. However, the IgG immunoglobulins were needed for ingestion and degradation of the target cells by the macrophages in reaction steps inhibitable by papain-digested fragments of IgG. In these experiments, IgM with or without cell-bound C3 mediated attachment but no ingestion. These experiments leave little doubt that processes such as phagocytosis, long considered solely as cellular phenomena, are markedly influenced by contributions of antibody and C from the serum.

Recent experiments in Dr. Nussenzweig's laboratory indicate that polymorphonuclear leukocytes and macrophages differ with respect to their C receptors, thereby influencing the rate and extent of phagocytosis. The polymorphonuclear leukocytes, like the erythrocytes, possess receptors for C3b and function through immune adherence. The monocytic phagocytes carry receptors for both C3b and its cleavage product C3d. Both of these C receptors participate in conjunction with IgG for the ingestion of sheep red blood cells.

The accumulated evidence therefore suggests that the functionally descriptive term "heat-labile opsonins" actually refers to conponents of the alternate C pathway as well as to specific or cross-reacting immunoglobulins present in minimal quantities in normal sera which are readily inactivated under the conventional thermal conditions.

The phagocytic process has been assigned a vital role in protecting the host against invasion by microorganisms which are impervious to the action of serum antibody and C and which can multiply in the cytoplasm of phagocytic cells after ingestion. Prominent examples include such pathogens as the staphylococci, virulent mycobacteria, listeria, and group A streptococci. The early studies of Lurie and the more recent work of Mackaness and his colleagues have emphasized important features of the interaction between these organisms and the host's monocytes. When these phagocytic cells are derived from a normal animal, they can ingest the organisms, but this process is followed by intracellular multiplication, cell destruction, and tissue death. When the phagocytic cells are furnished by a previously immunized animal, ingestion also takes place, but the invading pathogens are soon destroyed by the "activated" macrophages through liberation of their lysosomal enzymes. Moreover, activation of the macrophages does not follow immunization of the host with a vaccine containing dead organisms. This defense mechanism comes into play only after limited multiplication of the pathogen in the tissues. Since the passive administration of specific antibody does not influence the fate of the intracellular pathogens, the protective process which follows prior experience with living pathogens is considered to be cellular in nature, but little if at all affected by the humoral components of the immune response. The exclusion of antibody may not be absolute since prior experience with the same organism tips the scale from intracellular multiplication to intracellular degradation. Moreover, once activated by this immune event, the macrophages are capable of engulfing and destroying immunologically unrelated pathogens. Viewed in the context of the present discussion, it may not be implausible to suggest that humoral factors such as antibody and C may participate in the ingestion and intracellular destruction. Evidence for the acceleration of phagocytosis by antibody and C has been evaluated above. We need only add that recent studies, discussed in the next chapter, show that anaphylatoxins, products of C activation via the classical or properdin pathways, when present, lead to lysosomal enzyme release. This event could potentiate the enzymatic degradation of the intracellular parasite. In the absence of sufficient antibody, as may be the case with cells from normal animals, C activation may be minimal or lacking, thereby creating an environment suitable for intracellular multiplication.

Support for these speculative considerations may be drawn from experiments by Fudenberg and others which demonstrate specific receptor sites on human monocytes for IgG and C3. The date in Table 6-2 show that sheep erythrocytes are readily ingested by human monocytes when sensitized with IgG, or with the intermediate complex IgGC1423. IgM on

Table 6–2

Effect of C on ingestion by human monocytes of erythrocytes
sensitized with IgG or IgM antibody *

Erythrocyte complex	Addition to the medium	Monocytes with ingested red cells, %
EA(IgG)	None	94
EA(IgG)	IgG	6
EA(IgG)C1423	IgG	92
EA(IgM)	None	0
EA(IgM)	IgG	0
EA(IgM)C1423	None	18
EA(IgM)C1423	IgG	77

* Modified from H. Huber et al., *Science*, **162**:1282, 1968.

the red cells did not stimulate phagocytosis unless the designated C components were bound to the sensitized cells. Finally, the incorporation of IgG into the fluid phase of these reaction mixtures enhanced ingestion of those cells sensitized with IgMC1423 containing the immunoglobulin and C1,4,2,3.

The importance of the alternate pathway in mediating phagocytosis has been highlighted in studies of sickle-cell disease. As is known, patients with this abnormality are highly susceptible to bacterial infections, and particularly to pneumococcal meningitis. A recent estimation of the risk of infection of blacks with sickle-cell disease as compared to the total black population indicated that the chance of the former for contracting pneumococcal meningitis was 579 times greater than for the whites. Winkelstein and Drachman showed that the sera of sickle-cell patients failed to support phagocytosis of pneumococci, despite their normal levels of C1, C4, C2, and C3. The deficiency in phagocytosis was pinpointed to an inability of the sera of sickle-cell patients to utilize the alternate pathway as demonstrated by their feeble ability to opsonize zymosan particles or cleave C3 in this process.

VIRUS NEUTRALIZATION

The protective functions of the C system have been exemplified in two ways. Bacteriolysis requires completion of the sequence involving the classical or the alternate pathway, and the destructive process requires lysozyme. In phagocytosis, the presence of the proper intermediate in the C sequence permits the sensitized particle to perturb the membrane of the phagocytic cell so that ingestion is greatly accelerated. Studies of the role of C in virus neutralization have uncovered a third mechanism, namely, the binding of C components to sensitized virus particles in such a manner as to hinder the penetration of the target cell by the virion or otherwise interfere with virus replication. A striking example has recently been described by Adler and his associates. Inactivation of T2 bacteriophage by its antibody was increased a thousandfold when the virion-antibody complexes were formed in the presence of fresh normal, anti-immunoglobulin, or anti-allotype sera. This effect was observed only with immune sera obtained early in the course of immunizing rabbits with T2 phage. The enhancement was presumably achieved by enlarging the aggregate such as by the addition of C components, thereby minimizing dissociation and obstructing adsorption of the virus tail to the receptor on the membrane of the host cell. The degree of enhancement exerted by C is shown in Fig. 6-3.

The mechanism of virus neutralization enhancement by C has been clarified by studies in the laboratory of Rapp and Borsos. These investigators and their associates observed that the inactivation of sensitized herpes virus particles was markedly increased by the addition of purified C components. The major findings which confirmed reports published about twenty-five years ago and again more recently by Taniguchi and Yoshino are summarized in Fig. 6-4. As seen there, the efficacy of herpes virus neutralization varied with the concentration of antibody and the presence of C components in the reaction mixtures. In experiments with herpes virus sensitized with IgM antibody, the degree of virus inactivation varied directly with the concentration of C4, C2, or C3 when conditions were adjusted so that two of the three C components were in limited supply. An augmenting effect was noted with C4, C2, and C3, but not with the later-acting components, when relatively high antibody concentrations were used for sensitization. When the sensitizing antibody was decreased by a factor of 4 or 8, whole serum was more effective than the combined use of C4, C2, and C3. The binding of these components to the sensitized virion particles followed the same sequence as in immune hemolysis, i.e., an adequate supply of $C\bar{1}$ was needed to show the enhancing effects of C4, C2, or C3. The interpretation offered by these investigators was that the addition of C components hindered the attachment of the virions to the host cell. The addition of $C\bar{1}$ alone to the sensitized virus particles did not increase neutralization, probably because an insufficient number of cell sites were covered. With C4 and C3, the enhancing action could also be attributed to the amplification in the number of sites on the virion occupied by these components in the absence of $C\bar{1}$, such as the clustering effect noted in immune hemolytic studies.

Similar considerations probably apply to observations which demon-

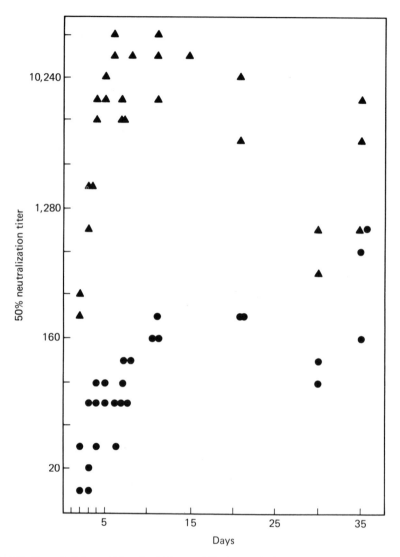

Fig. 6-3. T2 neutralizing activity of rabbit sera following a single intravenous injection of 10⁹ PFU T2 on day 0. Each symbol stands for the titer of one rabbit serum obtained on the day indicated. Assayed in the absence (●) or presence (▲) of 0.02 ml of active normal rat serum as complement source. PFU = plaque-forming units. (F. L. Adler, W. S. Walker, and M. Fishman, *Virology* **46**:800, 1971.)

strate the enhancement of virus neutralization which follows the binding of anti-immunoglobulins and rheumatoid factors to the sensitized virions. Since the publication of these reports, other examples of C-enhanced virus neutralization have been published. Enhanced neutralization of polyoma

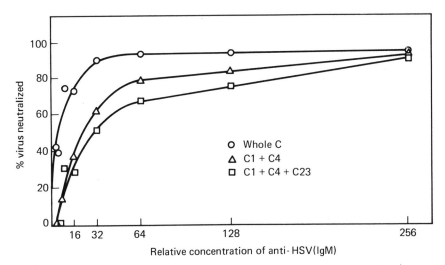

Fig. 6-4. Relationship between the concentration of antibody used to sensitize the virus and the amount of neutralization produced by whole guinea pig C and purified C components. Virus was sensitized with serial twofold dilutions of the IgM fraction of rabbit anti-HSV. Each preparation of HSV-IgM was reacted with optimal C1̄. Portions of 0.2 ml were removed and incubated for 30 min with equal volumes of C4 containing 6.0×10^{11} effective molecules/ml. The reaction mixtures were diluted with 0.4 ml of buffer. 0.3-ml portions were then removed from each reaction mixture and incubated for 30 min with 0.3 ml of either buffer or a mixture containing 6.0×10^{11} effective molecules of C2/ml and 3.0×10^{11} effective molecules of C3/ml. HSV-IgM which had been put through the same incubation and dilution steps but not exposed to C1̄, C4, C2, or C3 was incubated with undiluted whole guinea pig C. HSV = Herpes simplex virus. (C. A. Daniels, T. Borsos, H. J. Rapp, R. Snyderman, and A. L. Notkins, *Proc. Nat'l. Acad. Sci.*, **65**:534, 1970.)

virus-antibody complexes in the presence of C1, C4, C2, and C3 has also been demonstrated by Oldstone and others as shown in Table 6-3. Extrapolation of these observations to other infectious agents may not be amiss. One example which comes to mind is the action of immune serum in protecting rats from infection with the rodent malaria agent *P. berghei*. Diggs and the author demonstrated that passive immunization of rats with a specific antiserum delayed the onset and intensity of parasitemia. The effect was attributed to the inhibition of erythrocyte penetration by the merozoite form of the malaria parasite after sensitization by antibody. Under the *in vivo* conditions used in these experiments, it could be assumed that the binding of C components to the sensitized merozoites may have acted in a manner analogous to the action of C on the sensitized herpes virus. However, it was later shown that cobra venom treatment of rats infected with *P. berghei* had no effect on parasitemia levels so that the theoretical considerations have not yet been verified experimentally. Additional experiments involving restoration of the C deficiency with purified components seem indicated.

Table 6–3

Role of various C components in enhanced neutralization of
V-Ab complex *

Reagents added to virus-antibody mixture	% virus neutralization
Medium	0
Heated guinea pig serum	0
Normal guinea pig serum	86
C4-deficient guinea pig serum	0
Normal rabbit serum	73
C6-deficient rabbit serum	65
Normal human serum	80
Purified C1	0
Purified C1, C4	0
Purified C1, C4, C2	0
Purified C1, C4, C2, C3	84
Purified C1q	60

* From M. B. A. Oldstone, N. R. Cooper, and D. L. Larson, *J. Exp. Med.,* **140**:560, 1974.
For the polyoma plaque and neutralization assay stock polyoma virus was diluted and mixed
with a dilution of rabbit antibody to polyoma virus to give 50–55 PFU on confluent mouse embryo monolayers per 60 × 15 mm Falcon petri dish. All mixtures were diluted in Eagle's basic
medium and incubated at 37°C for 30 min.; a final vol of 0.2 ml was added to mid log Ha/ICR
embryo cells. PFU = Plaque forming units.

C RECEPTORS ON LYMPHOCYTES

Nussenzweig, Bianco, and their associates have opened a new avenue
of C research with the important observation that lymphocytes possess C
receptors, thereby implicating the C system in certain aspects of cellular
immunology. Their findings have been widely confirmed and extended in
the demonstration that other leukocytes in the monocytic series also possess
a variety of receptors for various C components. The role of these receptors
is under active study in attempts to evaluate the participation of membrane-
bound C components in the destruction of nucleated target cells through
the mediation of cellular immune processes. These receptors were demonstrated by the fact that sheep erythrocytes sensitized with Forsmann antibody formed rosettes on the lymphocyte surface in the presence of fresh
mouse serum. Lymphocytes of the mouse, rabbit, rat, guinea pig, and human possess these C receptors and have been called CRL (complement
receptor lymphocytes). A typical rosette formed with a mouse spleen
lymphocyte is shown in Fig. 6-5. Small- and medium-sized lymphocytes
present in the spleen and lymph nodes possess the C receptor and are
morphologically indistinguishable from other cells lacking the ability to
form rosettes with erythrocytes sensitized in the presence of serum. This
mechanism of rosette formation differs from the one involving the simple

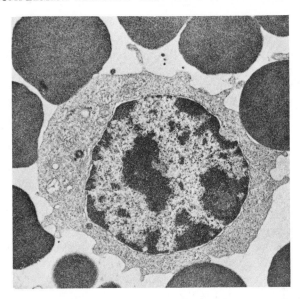

Fig. 6-5. A rosette of sensitized sheep erythrocytes adherent to a mouse spleen lymphocyte through its C receptor. (From L. T. Chen, A. Eden, V. Nussenzweig, and L. Weiss, *Cellular Immunology* 4:281, 1972.)

admixture of spleen lymphocytes with sheep erythrocytes. The latter has been attributed to thymus-derived lymphocytes which form red cell rosettes in the absence of added antibody or mouse serum as a source of C. The incidence of CRL varies in different mice but may be as high as 40% of the spleen lymphocytes. These cells are of bone-marrow origin and display their receptors when the erythrocytes are sensitized with 19S immunoglobulins and are in the state EAC423 or EAC43. Three different receptors have been identified in populations of peripheral lymphocytes and of cultured lymphoblastoid cells. Some cells bind only the Fc fragment of the immunoglobulins. A second group binds C3b, the C3 fragment which participates in immune adherence, while a third subpopulation binds C3d, the fragment of C3b which remains cell bound after cleavage by the C3 inactivator. A clear illustration for the presence of different receptors has been supplied by Shevach and others, who showed that lymphocytes of Balb/C mice with certain strains of leukemia possessed receptors for EA but not for EAC. The reverse situation was observed with lymphocytes of humans with chronic lymphocytic leukemia.

Fairly rigorous evidence has been provided for the involvement of C3 in the CRL. Thus, cells in the intermediate state of EAC4 do not form rosettes although Bokisch and others found C4 receptors on human B lymphocytes. The size and number of rosettes are directly proportional to the input of C3 into the reaction mixtures. Antibody to mouse C3 inhibits rosette formation and will, in fact, dissociate preformed rosettes. Cultured lymphocytes derived from a patient with Burkitt's lymphoma react similarly. Gelfand and co-workers found that the lymphocyte receptors for immunoglobulins arise during the first day of life, about two weeks prior to the appearance of C3b binding sites. Moreover, different strains of inbred mice vary in the number of lymphocytes which bear C receptors as shown in Fig. 6-6. Genetic studies by these investigators led them to surmise that one of the genes controlling the rate of CRL development is linked to the mouse H-2 complex. Genetic control of this characteristic was further demonstrated with lethally irradiated adult mice whose viability was restored with syngeneic bone-marrow cells. In these mice, the reappearance of CRL recapitulated the ontogeny of the cell donor.

The demonstration that some lymphocytes possess C3b as well as C3d receptors has naturally stimulated a number of inquiries as to their function. One area of study pertains to the hypothesis that the presence of these receptors on lymphocytes from tumor-bearing animals might possibly enhance the cytotoxic action of these "killer" cells for neoplastic cells. Studies in several laboratories failed to detect any influence of C components or pathways in the destruction of target cells by sensitized lymphocytes. However, G. Möller has recently proposed that, when the target cells are sensitized with both Fc fragments and C3, they are more susceptible to the

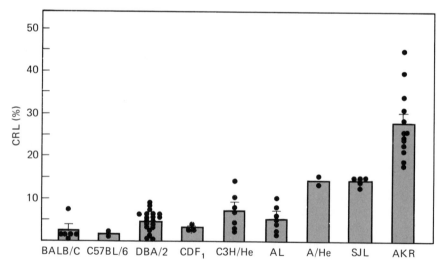

Fig. 6-6. Percent of lymphocytes bearing C receptors, as determined by rosette formation, in spleens of 2-wk old mice of various strains. (From M. C. Gelfand, G. V. Elfenbein, M. M. Frank, and W. E. Paul, *J. Exp. Med.*, **139**:1129, 1974.)

cytotoxic action of sensitized lymphocytes. This greater vulnerability was not apparent when the target cells carried only the immunoglobulin Fc fragments or C3. It is pertinent to note in this context that Osther and Dybkjaer found Clq, C4, C3 and C3 Activator ($\overline{B}$) on 10 to 25% of human lymphocytes.

ANTIBODY SYNTHESIS

A second area currently under active investigation concerns the role of C3 lymphocyte receptors in antibody synthesis. Positive evidence of this has been contributed by several laboratories. Thus Diamantstein, Battisto, and their co-workers demonstrated an increase in hemolytic plaque-forming cells in mice injected with dextran sulfate after having been irradiated, injected with syngeneic bone marrow cells, and immunized with sheep red blood cells. The nonspecific enhancement of antibody production was also observed by Coutinho and Möller and has been linked to the capacity of substances such as dextran sulfate and other polyanions to substitute for thymus-dependent lymphocytes through activation of the alternate pathway. This deduction was drawn to explain the fact that certain antigens like pneumococcal polysaccharides and bacterial lipopolysaccharides, which can also trigger the alternate C system, stimulate antibody synthesis without the cooperation of thymus-derived lymphocytes. The C involvement in these events was strengthened by the report of M. B. Pepys who showed that *in vivo* depletion of C3 by cobra venom factor was associated with suppression of hemagglutinating antibodies to sheep erythrocytes (Fig. 6-7) but not to pneumococcal polysaccharides. He considered that the fixation of C3 on the C receptors of lymphocytes augmented the binding and processing of antigen by macrophages and thereby increased antibody production. Analogous results were obtained when spleen cells of immunized mice were cultured in the presence of antibody to mouse C3. Secondary responses to a thymus-dependent immunogen were suppressed, whereas antibody formation to a thymus-independent antigen was unaffected. Subsequent studies by Janossy and co-workers led to the more restricted conclusion that C3 participates in the thymus-dependent immune response as an auxiliary factor by increasing cooperation between thymus and bone-marrow-derived lymphocytes rather than as an essential mitogen for the latter cells. In evaluating the available evidence, Dukor and Hartmann concluded that antibody-secreting cells could be activated by two means. One mechanism involves the specific binding of antigens by immunoglobulin receptors on lymphocytes. A second involves activation of the alternate pathway by compounds like dextran sulphate and the union of C3b with the C receptor on bone-marrow-derived lymphocytes.

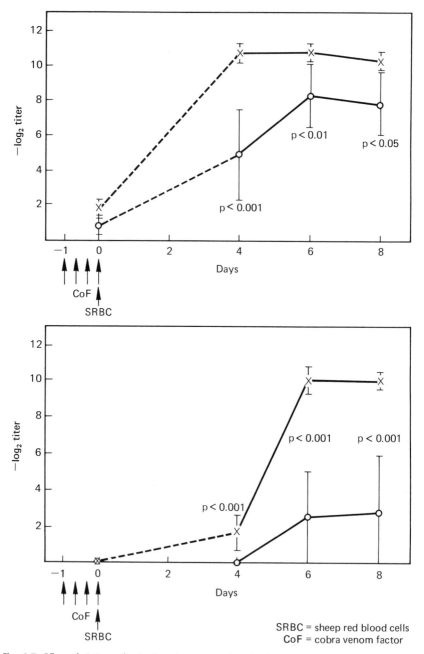

Fig. 6-7. Effect of CoF on the total and mercaptoethanol-resistant anti-SRBC response. CoF was given to the test animals so as to produce maximal depletion of circulating C3 between 2–4 days after intraperitoneal injection of 2.5×10^8 SRBC. Above, total antibody titers; below, mercapto-ethanol-resistant antibody titers.   X = controls treated with phosphate-buffered saline; O = CoF treated mice; arrow indicates interperitoneal injection. (From M. B. Pepys, *J. Exp. Med.,* **140**:129, 1974.)

A somewhat different interpretation of the suppressive effect of cobra factor on antibody synthesis has been proposed by Nielsen and White. They observed that, after treatment with the cobra factor, a single, rather large injection of sheep erythrocytes into chickens (10^{10} cells per bird) resulted in a cyclical appearance of hemagglutinating antibodies. When the birds were not treated with cobra venom factor, there was a slight diminution in the initial antibody level, but no recurrent elevations were observed, as shown in Fig. 6-8. As judged by the criterion of destructability by 0.3 M 2-mercaptoethanol, much of the antibody in the treated birds was of the 19S class. Moreover, the chickens treated with cobra factor produced no 7S immunoglobulins. Nielsen and White suggest that cobra venom factor converts the normal response to a thymus-dependent antigen (sheep erythrocytes) into one characteristic of a thymus-indifferent antigen. The latter, they propose, fails to switch 19S to 7S antibody production and does not induce a homeostatic termination of the immune response because it ac-

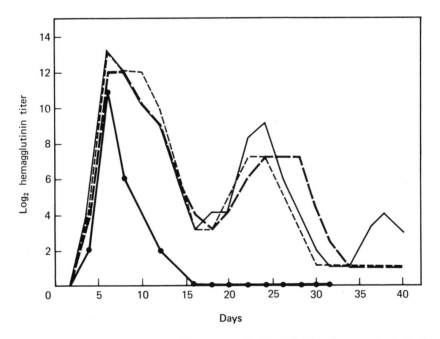

Fig. 6-8. Anti-sheep RBC response in chickens treated with CoF. Plot of hemagglutinin levels (log$_2$ titer) following an intravenous injection of 10^{10} sheep erythrocytes. ●———● The average hemagglutinin titers for a group of 10 normal birds. The response reaches maximum at 6 d and thereafter rapidly declines, remaining at or near zero after 16 d. ——— , --- , —— — , Hemagglutinin titers of individual birds treated with cobra venom factor (CoF). The first hemagglutinin response of all birds is slightly increased in comparison with controls at the peak and delayed in the decline phase; all birds also show a further peak (maximum at day 24–25). In the case of one bird a further (third) peak developed (maximum at day 38). (From K. H. Nielsen, and R. G. White, *Nature* **250**:234, 1974.)

tivates the alternate pathway, thereby converting C3 to its inactive degradation product.

It is apparent that these findings have enlarged the scope of C research, and it may be anticipated that clarifying data will soon become available to permit a more precise evaluation of the role of the C system in the complex process leading to antibody synthesis.

FURTHER READING

Daniel, C. A., Borsos, T., Rapp., H. J., Snyderman, R., and Notkins, A. L., "Neutralization of Sensitized Virus by Purified Components of Complement," *Proc. Nat'l Acad. Sci.*, **65**:528, 1970.

Davis, S. D., Gemsa, D., and Wedgwood, R. J., "Kinetics of the Transformation of Gram-Negative Rods to Spheroplasts and Ghosts by Serum," *J. Immunol.*, **96**:570, 1966.

Diamantstein, T., Meinhold, H., and Wagner, B., "Stimulation of Humoral Antibody Formation by Polyanions," *Eur. J. Immunol.*, **1**:429, 1971, and earlier papers.

Dukor, P., and Hartmann, K. U., "Bound C3 as a Second Signal for B-Cell Activation," *Cellular Immunol.*, **7**:349, 1973.

Gelfand, M. C. et al., "Ontogeny of B Lymphocytes," *J. Exp. Med.*, **139**:1125, 1974.

Glynn, A. A., and Howard, C. J., "The Sensitivity to Complement of Strains of *Escherichia coli* Related to their K Antigens," *Immunology*, **18**:331, 1970.

Inoue, K., Yonemasu, K., Takamizawa, A., and Amano, T., "Requirement of All Nine Components of Complement for Immune Bacteriolysis," *Biken Journal*, **11**:203, 1968, and earlier papers.

Janossy, G., Humphrey, J. H., Pepys, M. B., and Greaves, M. F., "Complement Independence of Stimulation of Mouse Splenic B Lymphocytes by Mitogens," *Nature New Biol.*, **245**:108, 1973.

Nelson, D. S., "Immune Adherence," *Advances in Immunology.*, **3**:131, 1963.

Nelson, R. A. Jr., "The Immune Adherence Phenomenon," *Science*, **118**:733, 1953.

Nussenzweig, V., "Receptors for Immune Complexes on Lymphocytes," *Advances in Immunology*, **19**:217, 1974.

Oldstone, M. B. A., Cooper, N. R., and Larson, D. L., "Formation and Biologic Role of Polyoma Virus—Antibody Complexes: A critical role for Complement," *J. Exp. Med.*, **140**:549, 1974.

Pepys, M. B., "Role of Complement in Induction of Antibody Production *in Vivo*," *J. Exp. Med.,* **140**:126, 1974.

Ross, G. D. and Polley, M. J., "Specificity of Human Lymphocyte Complement Receptors," *J. Exp. Med.* **141**:1163, 1975.

Chapter 7

Additional Aspects of

Complement-mediated Cytotoxicity

Knowledge of the sequential component reactions which culminate in immune hemolysis, as described in Chapters 2 and 3, has been applied in studies of leukocyte and platelet destruction by antibody and C. A description of these events and some *in vivo* C functions involving the formed blood elements are discussed in this chapter. It is obviously more difficult to delineate the individual reaction steps or identify the intermediates of the classical or alternate C pathways under *in vivo* conditions. Nevertheless, considerable information is available at both the theoretical and experimental levels which strengthens the conviction that the sequences outlined in the earlier chapters, based on *in vitro* experiments, faithfully reflect the mechanisms of cell destruction by antibody and C in the tissues.

IMMUNE HEMOLYSIS IN VIVO

Forssman Shock

This term is applied to the sequence which follows the intravenous injection of Forssman antiserum into animals like the guinea pig, whose tissues contain the heterophile or Forssman antigen. Within minutes, a succession of symptoms are noted which includes intense coughing, nose-scratching, ruffling of the furry coat, the appearance of a blood-tinged nasal exudate, and death due to extensive and hemorrhagic pulmonary edema. The hemorrhagic events are undoubtedly due to red cell lysis initiated by interaction of the erythrocytes with the Forssman antibody and activation of the classical pathway as indicated in Chapter 2. Since guinea pig tissues other than the red cells also contain the Forssman glycolipid, the other symptoms, like the nose-scratching and edema, may probably be attributed to the local release of anaphylatoxins and other vasoactive agents as discussed in the next chapter. The analogy between the Forssman shock and immune hemolysis *in vitro* is sustained by the observations in C4-deficient guinea pigs. When the deficiency is absolute, as in homozygous animals, the injection of Forssman antibody is without effect. The passive administration of purified C4 several hours prior to the antiserum renders the deficient animals susceptible to Forssman shock, but death does not occur in the reconstituted animals for several hours. The delay may simply reflect the time needed for the C4 to be distributed to the extravascular compartments, such as the pulmonary tissues, which are the major sites of the fatal edema. The mechanistic differences between systemic anaphylaxis due to IgE and Forssman shock due to IgG or IgM are apparent. Although respiratory distress occurs in both instances, reagin-mediated anaphylaxis is readily produced in C4-deficient guinea pigs and without signs of hemorrhage. In contrast, the rapidity of the Forssman shock evolution has been correlated with the available amount of C4 to the animal. Whereas fatal reactions occur within a minute or two in normal guinea pigs with C4 titers of 50,000 hemolytic units per milliliter, death is delayed for several minutes in heterozygous animals with C4 titers in the range of 5500 to 18,000, while guinea pigs with an absolute deficiency of C4 are indifferent to the injection of Forssman antibody.

HEMOLYSIS MEDIATED BY C AND "AUTOANTIBODIES"

This heading encompasses red cell destruction associated with a variety of clinical conditions prominent among which are bacterial, fungal, and viral infections, hemolytic anemias associated with antibiotic and drug therapy, as well as situations involving antibody responses to autologous or isologous antigens. This simple statement of the phenomenon is itself indicative of the multiplicity of antigenic determinants which can initiate the so-called autoimmune hemolytic anemias, and the resulting diversity of the immune responses with respect to antibody class. It is therefore to be expected that, in some of these situations, the erythrocytes may contain immunoglobulins on their surfaces which fail to activate the C system. Such cells may, however, be cleared from the circulation by phagocytosis or sequestration.

With respect to the participation of C, several mechanisms may be operative. A likely one is based on the notion that the low molecular weight agent used for therapeutic purposes, or antigenic determinants liberated from the infectious agents or their metabolically degraded products, become bound to host tissue constituents either as complete antigens or in a manner analogous to the formation of hapten-protein conjugates. The binding which occurs *in vivo* need not be covalent in nature to initiate an immune response. Some of the immunoglobulins formed as a result of this stimulation will be specific for the microbial agent, the drug, or the antibiotic. The binding of these determinants to a red cell or platelet membrane in the presence of specific antibody and C reproduces the conditions favoring passive hemolysis or thrombocytolysis via either of the C pathways. The immunologic consequences of penicillin therapy provide a pertinent and well-studied example.

A second mechanism which may be implicated in these events pertains to the formation of immunogenic determinants on erythrocytes which have bound fragmented C components such as C3b or C3d. These cells are vulnerable to erythrophagocytosis, agglutination or lysis through the synthesis of specific antibodies or immunoconglutinins. The antibody class involved is varied. Most commonly they are of the IgG class, although many reports implicate the IgM antibodies such as those identified as "cold-agglutinins." Secretory IgA antibodies have also been identified in C-dependent erythrophagocytosis.

Rosse has used the $\overline{C1}$ transfer reaction of Borsos and Rapp to determine the number of IgG molecules on red cells from patients with immune hemolytic anemia. Estimates of cell-bound IgM present no serious problem since a single antibody molecule activates C1. Enumeration of $\overline{C1}$ molecules transferred from the erythrocytes treated with monospecific anti-IgM to EAC4 therefore yields a minimal value for the number of IgM molecules per cell. In experiments with guinea pig erythrocytes sensitized *in vivo* with rabbit IgM immunoglobulins, Schreiber and Frank estimated that as few as sixty C-fixing sites per cell were needed for accelerated clearance. The procedure for IgG is somewhat more involved. The difficulty stems from the fact that the fixation of a single molecule of $\overline{C1}$ requires at least two molecules of IgG in an appropriate topographic configuration. To fulfill this condition, about 2000 molecules of IgG antibody seem to be required. However, if all the cell-bound IgG used to sensitize the cells were properly disposed in the form of doublets, a simple correction factor could be applied, but nature is rarely so compliant. Consequently, experimental conditions have to be adjusted with respect to cell number, the antibody (in the serum of a patient with hemolytic anemia), the anti-IgG reagent (prepared in goats or rabbits), and the amount of C1 added so that the uptake of this component will be directly proportional to the amount of anti-IgG. As suggested by Borsos and Rapp earlier, Rosse standardized these conditions so that log-log plots yield a linear relationship between the number of $\overline{C1}$ molecules fixed and the relative serum concentrations. Graphs of results obtained with IgM and IgG antibodies are shown in Fig. 7-1. In repetitive assays of one human serum,

---

Fig. 7-1. Logarithmic dose-response plots for the titration of IgM (autoimmune cold agglutinin, upper panel) and IgG (autoimmune warm agglutinin, lower panel) as a function of the number of $\overline{C1}$ molecules bound per 10^3 human erythrocytes. (From W. F. Rosse, *J. Clin. Investigation,* **47:**2440, 1968.)

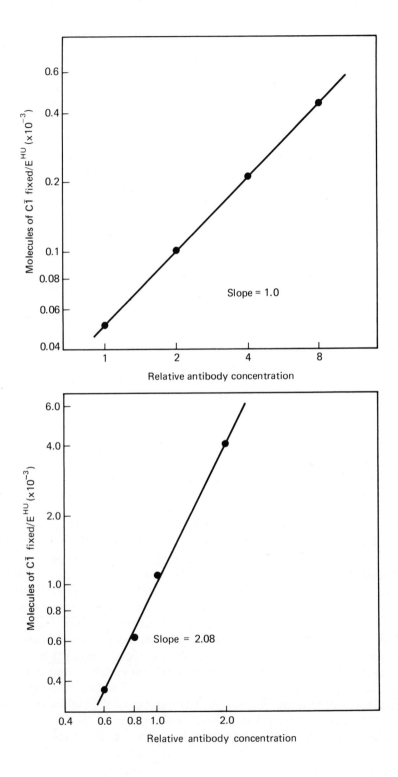

the number of activated $C\overline{1}$ molecules per cell ranged between 1020 and 1310. In similar assays with the serum of a patient containing anti-D immunoglobulins, the number ranged from 3850 to 6380. With other Rh antigens, the cell surface distribution was evidently too sparse to permit the formation of enough doublets capable of fixing detectable numbers of $C\overline{1}$.

The *in vivo* implications of these studies have also been evaluated by Rosse, who assayed cell-bound and "warm" antibody levels in sera from patients with autoimmune hemolytic anemia associated with chronic lymphocytic leukemia, systemic lupus, idiopathic thrombocytopenic purpura, etc. The cell-bound antibody assays were performed with the patients' red cells, anti-IgG, and C1. Cells from healthy donors were pre-incubated with the patients' sera prior to admixture with anti-IgG and C1. The results showed that the degree of *in vivo* hemolysis was generally related to the level of cell-bound antibody. Both parameters decreased after splenectomy, as shown in Fig. 7-2.

Prednisone therapy diminishes the levels of cell-bound antibody with concomitant increases in serum concentrations and symptomatic relief. With continued drug administration and remission, serum antibody levels were also lowered. In view of the degree of *in vivo* hemolysis, activation of the classical pathway would seem to account for the anemia, although participation of the alternate pathway of C activation is not necessarily excluded. The presence of $C\overline{1}$ or other C components on red cell membranes does not necessarily result in lysis but does lead to shortened survival times. Okada and his colleagues reported a significant increase in electrophoretic mobility of sheep red cells in the states $EAC\overline{142}$ and $EAC\overline{1423}$. These findings are in keeping with those of Mardiney and others who used ferritin-labeled antisera to C4 and C3 to detect membrane-bound components. Cells containing the early C intermediates with 450 C4 molecules per erythrocyte were able to degrade 100,000 molecules of C3. Although not all of the bound C3 need propagate the lytic reaction, the membranes are altered and become more vulnerable to phagocytosis and sequestration. Evidence along these lines has been provided by Logue, Rosse, and Gockerman in their studies of patients with the cold agglutinin syndrome. Evans and co-workers, as well as others, had earlier demonstrated low serum C in patients with these immunoglobulins. Logue and others carried the investigation further through assays of cell-bound C3 with anti-C3 by means of the $C\overline{1}$ transfer reaction. When patients were subjected to cold stress with the production of intravascular hemolysis, cell-bound C3 levels in one patient were almost doubled within ten minutes, as judged by their capacity to bind $C\overline{1}$. The number of $C\overline{1}$ molecules bound to the C3-anti-C3 complexes was directly proportional to the C3 content of the cells. The dependence of *in vivo* hemolysis on the number of C3

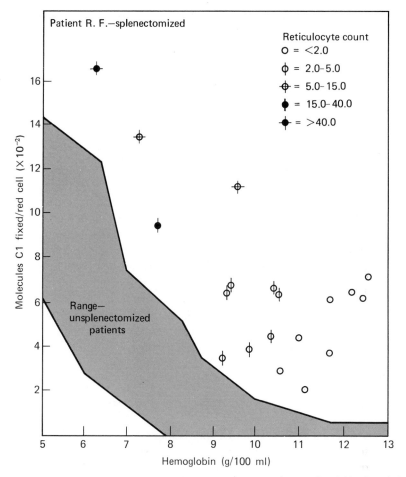

Fig. 7-2. The relationship between hemoglobin concentration in the peripheral blood and the concentration of cell-bound antibody in patient R. F. who had undergone splenectomy. The range for unsplenectomized patients is shown in the shaded area. The patient was taking 0–10 mg of prednisone at the time of the determinations. (From W. F. Rosse, *J. Clin. Investigation,* **50**:738, 1971.)

molecules per cell has been confirmed in studies of hemolytic anemia by Fischer and his co-workers. They reported that overt hemolysis occurred in eight of eleven patients whose red cells carried more than 1100 molecules of C3 per cell. With a lower burden of C3 only two of fourteen patients had demonstrable hemolytic anemia. Further studies of this type should be more generally applicable to a variety of cytopathic events, particularly since monospecific antisera to several of the C components have become available. As described in Chapter 4, Borsos and Leonard have recently described another technique to estimate cell-attached or fluid-phase C3 by adding the test material to a reference anti-C3 serum and then measuring the degree of lysis of sheep EC3 in the presence of whole guinea pig C.

HEMOLYSIS MEDIATED BY C IN THE APPARENT ABSENCE OF ANTIBODY (PAROXYSMAL NOCTURNAL HEMOGLOBINURIA, PNH)

Red cells of patients with this disorder are highly susceptible to lysis by C in the apparent absence of an exogenous antibody source. These cells also undergo spontaneous lysis in slightly acidified serum. Moreover, when they are incubated in serum at pH = 8.0 together with cobra venom factor, irreversible membrane damage ensues. Normal red cells mimic the susceptibility of PNH erythrocytes when treated with reduced glutathione. Recent experiments demonstrated that the lysis of PNH cells in inulin-serum mixtures was mediated through the C3 proactivator, i.e., the precursor of the C3-cleaving enzyme in the alternate pathway. These results are consistent with the earlier demonstration of a properdin requirement for this reaction. The intervention of the classical pathway in the lysis of these cells establishes their vulnerability to either of the C-activation mechanisms. Since the PNH cells show a relatively greater uptake of C5 than C3, it has been speculated that lysis takes place through the generation and activity of the short-lived intermediate C567 as in reactive lysis.

LYSIS OF NUCLEATED CELLS BY ANTIBODY AND C

Several recent reports describe the fixation of C components, with or without ensuing lysis, by virus-transformed cells and antiviral antibody. These studies bear on the ability of the host's immune response to effect destruction of tumor cells *in vivo* through the mediation of C and antibody to the virus that initiates malignant transformation. Cikes found that cytotoxicity of virus-transformed murine lymphoma cells by antiviral antibody is dependent not only on the level of specific immunoglobulins but also on the growth phase of the cells. Sensitivity to cytolysis was greatest during the G1 phase of cell growth, presumably due to the extent of gene expression with respect to the density, distribution, and availability on the membrane of the viral antigens capable of binding specific antibody and activating C. An extension of Cikes' findings has been provided by the experiments of Lerner and others working with an antiserum to Moloney sarcoma virus and mouse cells. This antiserum was not reactive with normal mouse cells. As did Cikes, these authors found that cells in the logarithmic growth phase were less susceptible to C lysis despite their capacity to bind various C components as shown by the data in Table 7-1.

Table 7–1

Consumption of C components on addition of antiviral antibody
and serum by a synchronized population of mouse lymphoma
(YCAB) cells *

Time after release from G1, phase (hr)	Phase of cell cycle †	Percent of C component consumed in presence of antiviral antibody §						Cytotoxicity %
		C2	C3	C4	C5	C8	C9	
0	Early G_1	38	67	36	31	38	64	>50
5	Late G_1	38	59	32	17	30	53	<50
11	S	38	67	36	31	38	64	0
23	S, G_2, M	38	67	40	35	38	67	0
	M ‡		70					0

* From Lerner et al., Proc. Nat. Acad. Sci., **68:**2587, 1971.
† Viral antigen present on at least 50% of the cells in all growth stages.
‡ Arrested in metaphase by colcemid.
§ Immunoelectrophoretic studies showed that incubation of the cells with antibody and C activated the alternate pathway in terms of C3 proactivator conversion to C3A.

These findings and those based on fluorescence and electron microscopy and immune adherence assays revealed the presence of viral antigens, C5, C8, and even ultrastructural lesions on the cell membranes during the S, G_2 and M phases of cell growth without cytotoxicity. In the presence of viral antibody, activation of the classical and alternate pathways was also observed. The lack of cytotoxicity in stages other than G1 was therefore not attributable to absence of the antigen-antibody-C interaction, but to other factors which merit further study.

An important variable which governs C activation during various stages of the cell cycle concerns the nature of the target cell. Thus, Pellegrino and his co-workers found that the RPM 18866 line of cultured human lymphoid cells vary in their susceptibility to lysis by rabbit, human, and guinea pig C. However, the varied lytic susceptibility was not dependent upon the density of the HL-A antigens on these cells nor upon their ability to bind radio-labeled C components. These investigators concluded that the variable cytotoxicity might be attributed to changes in the cell membrane structure or the capacity of the cells to repair C-dependent membrane lesions. Another variable to be considered in studies of this type has been indicated by Basch. This investigator observed that the presence of non-C-fixing immunoglobulins in some alloantisera used for the cytotoxicity experiments can reduce the effective concentration of antigen on the target cell, thereby lowering the extent of cell destruction.

The question naturally arises in a discussion of these experiments as to the role of the classical and alternate pathways in the destruction of nucleated cells by antibody and C. May and his associates attacked this problem with several immune systems utilizing conventional and C4-deficient guinea pig sera as C sources. As indicated by the data in Table 7-2, the participation of the properdin system was negligible as judged by the feeble efficiency of the C4-deficient serum to mediate this antibody-dependent cytotoxic reaction. In view of the interrelationships between the classical and properdin pathways as envisioned by the experiments of Brade and others, the data shown in Table 7-2 will undoubtedly be sub-

Table 7–2

Cytotoxicity of normal and C4D serum for sensitized nucleated cells expressed as percent ^{51}Cr release *

	Antibody dilutions	Normal serum	C4D ‖ serum
Burro anti-T cell antibody versus	1:10	79.8	0 †
guinea pig thymus cells	1:64	75.0	— ‡
	1:128	66.0	—
	1:256	46.0	—
Mouse anti-θ C3H antibody versus	1:6	82.8 §	20.6 §
BALB/c thymus cells	1:12	—	27.5
	1:24	—	16.7
	1:48	—	15.1
	1:96	—	14.8
	1:100	77.7	—
	1:1000	70.4	—
	1:2000	63.1	—
	1:4000	63.6	—
	1:6000	65.8	—
Guinea pig strain 2 histocompatibil-	1:5	60	0
ity antibody versus L₂C guinea pig	1:10	53	0
leukemia cells	1:20	36	0
	1:40	7	0
	1:80	0	0

* From May, Green, and Frank, J. Immunol., **109**:599, 1972.
† No ^{51}Cr release.
‡ Not determined.
§ Obtained in a second experiment.
‖ C4D refers to serum from C4-deficient guinea pigs.

jected to further study. The experiments of Koene and McKenzie illustrate several facets of this problem. These investigators studied the actions of allo- and heteroantisera to the L1210 leukemia strain in DBA/2 mice. In reaction systems with limited antibody, rabbit serum C was far more effective than that of the guinea pig. With an excess of antibody, the two sera were equally effective. While these findings may not relate directly to the issue of alternate pathway activity in the cytolysis of nucleated mammalian cells, they do illustrate the fact that relatively minor changes in protocol may markedly influence the outcome of C-dependent reactions. In the present instance, it may be noted that the ratio of guinea pig to rabbit C activities in immune hemolysis approximates 15. More direct evidence of alternate pathway activity in the lysis of nucleated mammalian cells emerges from experiments with the Raji cell line derived from a patient with Burkitt lymphoma. These cells are lysed in a medium containing fresh normal human serum and cobra venom factor. They contain a receptor for C3b but do not participate in immune adherence, suggesting that the C3d fragment is not the binding site. Since lysis was prevented by inactivation of C3PA (Factor B) and required C6, intervention of the alternate pathway in this process was thereby deduced. Ferrone and colleagues evaluated the destruction of human lymphocytes by alloantibodies and human C. A marked variability was observed in the sense that some antisera activated C either through the classical or alternate pathway while others utilized C only when both pathways were involved. The data in Table 7-3 summarizes these findings.

Table 7-3

Evidence for mediation of a lymphocytotoxic reaction with HL-A alloantisera through the alternate and/or classical pathways of human complement *

Treatment of complement source	Cytolytic activity involving		
	Alternate pathway	Classical pathway	Both pathways
Control	+	+	+
C3PA-depleted	0	ND †	+
C3PA-depleted + C3PA	+	ND	+
Heated 50°C/20 min	0	+	+
Heated 50°C/20 min + C3PA	+	ND	+
C2-deficient	+	0	+
C2-deficient + C2	+	+	+
EGTA-treated	+	0	+
EDTA-treated	0	0	0

* From Ferrone, S., Cooper, N. R., Pellegrino, M. A., and Reisfeld, R. A., *Transplantation Proc.*, 6:16, 1974.
† ND = not done.

ALLOGRAFT REACTIONS

The participation of C as a decisive factor in the rejection of transplants from allogeneic hosts remains a matter of conjecture. As indicated above, nucleated cells subjected to the action of antibody in the presence of C are vulnerable to destruction through cytolysis or sequestration. However, the significance of these events in the rejection of solid tissue grafts cannot be adequately evaluated at present, particularly in terms of the current view that cell-mediated phenomena are independent of the C system and the difficulty in sorting out the humoral and cellular immune factors in these complex events. Certain facts have been established. These include the well-founded observations of humoral antibody formation following allogeneic transplants in man and other animals. The C-activating potencies of these immunoglobulins have not been carefully evaluated. Indeed it has been shown, following the work of Kaliss with mouse tumors, that in some instances specific immunoglobulins may exert an enhancing effect on tumor growth and cell survival. There are a number of observations which point to the need for further study of the interrelationships between humoral and cellular events and the competing effects of different immuno-globulin classes in promoting graft rejection. Drs. T. and S. Harris have shown that diminution of the gamma-1 immunoglobulin levels in mice prolongs the survival of allogeneic transplants.

The clearest demonstrations of graft rejection by antibody and C stem from the use of xenografts since the rejection process in these instances is more acute and intense. The use of xenografts to elucidate the mechanisms of transplantation immunity may be subject to the criticism that this experimental model does not faithfully reflect the intricate processes presumed to govern the rejection of allografts.

The data obtained in the course of studies such as reported by Winn and others are also very pertinent. In these experiments, rat ear skin was grafted onto adult mice which had previously been thymectomized and injected repeatedly with rabbit antiserum to mouse lymphocytes. Under these conditions, the grafts became well vascularized and viable. About two weeks after transplantation, the mice were injected with various reagents to determine their effect on graft survival. The median survival time for the rat ear skin was 7.8 days on normal mice and 31.6 days on the mice subjected to thymectomy and depletion of their immunocompetent cells. In the latter group, signs of graft damage were evident within 10 minutes and the grafts were rejected within 24–48 hours after the injection of a mouse anti-rat serum. The C system was implicated in the rejection process since depletion of C by the injection of cobra venom or heat-aggregated gamma globulin into the mice bearing the xenografts delayed or abrogated the rejection induced by mouse anti-rat serum. The use of a C5-deficient mouse strain (B10.D2 old) was also instructive. In 32 such mice injected with varying volumes of the mouse anti-rat serum, 16 failed to reject the ear skin for 2 to 5 weeks, as compared to only 3 transplants which survived in 44 B10.D2 new mice whose sera contained C5. In the C5-positive mice, 41 of the 44 recipients of the rat antiserum lost their grafts within 3–5 days. The activities of polymorphonuclear cells were also deemed essential for the rejection process which was thought to be initiated in the vascular endothelium. These experiments supplement the detailed studies of Cinader and others which showed that antilymphocyte serum exerts a dual effect, i.e., immunosuppression and graft-retention activity. The extent of the latter was C5-dependent, as demonstrated by comparing graft survival in co-isogenic C5-deficient and C5-competent mice. Analogies between these events and the induction of Arthus-type immune vasculitis will be discussed in Chapter 9.

Several additional reports support the interpretation that the constellation of immunologic processes which accompany the rejection of transplanted tissues includes utilization of the C system. The Rothers observed that destruction of the allograft, sarcoma I tumor cells, in B10.D2 old line mice (C5-deficient) proceeded with about one-tenth the efficiency of the rejection process in the co-isogenic B10.D2 new line animals (C5-positive). Interestingly, the tumor cells bound mouse globulins and C3 within minutes after inoculation.

The alternate pathway has been implicated in allograft survival by Pepys, who found that repeated injections of cobra venom within a well-defined period vis-a-vis transplantation of the graft retarded the rejection process. In experiments of this type, the delay due to C depletion may simply reflect interference with the inflammatory process surrounding the allograft.

The fundamental question that arises in the interpretation of these observations pertains to the need for C in the rejection process, i.e., in the destruction of the transplanted cells required for graft survival. Some support for the participation of C in cytotoxic processes mediated by leukocytes has been provided by Perlmann and his colleagues. It was observed that sensitized chicken erythrocytes bearing human C1,4,2,3 or C1,4,2,3,5,6,7 were slowly destroyed (60–80%) after 14 hours, as judged by the release of ^{51}Cr from the target cells. Target cells bearing C3 in either of the two complexes released the radiolabel after incubation with monocytes. Lymphocytes attacked only those cells in the state EAC1-3.

In subsequent studies, they found that ^{51}Cr-labeled chicken erythrocytes bearing C5, C6, and C7 released the isotope marker through the process of reactive lysis upon the addition of C8 and C9. The chicken erythrocytes in the state EC567 were also lysed by the addition of extensively washed human blood lymphocytes. The latter reaction was dependent upon the presence of C8 which was provided by the well-washed lymphocytes. Nonliving lymphocytes were equally effective in this reaction which could be abrogated by the addition of anti-C8. In contrast to these findings, the destruction of antibody-coated target cells, e.g., EA, apparently proceeds without the intervention of the terminal C components. Thus, the

Perlmanns and Lachmann have shown that, whereas the $F(ab')_2$ dimer of an anti-C8 serum abolishes the reactive lysis of E567 by C8, this reagent has no effect on the destruction of EA by lymphocytes. These findings suggest that a complement-dependent cytotoxic process accompanies graft rejection.

However experiments pertaining to the destruction of target cells by lymphocytes furnished by a specifically immunized animal have failed to detect a role for C. Henney and Mayer were unable to diminish the extent of ^{51}Cr release from mastocytoma cells by immune lymphocytes upon the addition of antisera to C2, C3, or C5. Other investigators also failed to observe any evidence for C in the lysis of antibody-coated erythrocytes by immune lymphocytes.

PLATELET LYSIS BY C AND ANTIBODY

The immune destruction of platelets has been studied extensively to clarify an important mechanism of C action and to enlarge our understanding of thrombocytopenia as a clinical entity. We can readily distinguish three types of immune platelet injury. The first, with which we will not be concerned, ensues from agglutination of these cells by specific antibody directed towards the viscous platelet membrane or to antigenic determinants adhering to the membrane. The latter may be derived from C components, plasma constituents resulting from blood coagulation, infectious agents, etc.

The other two mechanisms are both C- and antibody-dependent. In one type, the specificity of the antibody is directed towards constituents of the platelet membrane or to other antigenic determinants attached to the membranes of these cells. The second concerns an allergic type of platelet lysis by C and an unrelated immune system.

Antiplatelet Antibody

There is little reason to suppose that the modes of interaction of antiplatelet antibody with platelets and C differ from that of immune hemolysis or immune C-dependent cytotoxicity in general. Indeed, experiments carried out by Dr. Gocke in the author's laboratory established the overall similarities between the immune release of hemoglobin from sensitized erythrocytes and the release of histamine from specifically sensitized rabbit platelets by C. Considerable attention has been paid, however, to the immunologic aspects of thrombocytopenia in humans following relatively prolonged administration of certain drugs. Quinidine and Sedormid seem to be the most frequent culprits, although a number of other drugs have been incriminated in this regard. Antibodies to these agents have been demonstrated in the sera of many patients with drug-induced thrombocyto-penia. The action of these drugs as immunogens has been established by Shulman who demonstrated the *in vivo* destruction of platelets by admin-istering the incriminated drug or antiplatelet isoantibody to patients receiv-ing the specific drug.

Shulman postulated that the drug acts as a hapten which combines with noncellular plasma constituents or with the platelets. The antibody formed in response to the drug-macromolecule complex can then destroy platelets to which the drug has adhered. He also demonstrated that the *in vivo* lysis of platelets under these conditions with 4×10^{-9} M quinidine exceeds, by several orders of magnitude, the sensitivity of *in vitro* C-fixation assays with these reagents, which is inapparent at 10^{-6} M of this drug, as shown in Fig. 7-3.

The difference in sensitivity between these two immune manifestations is fully in accord with the principle outlined in Chapter 4, namely, for a given weight of immune complex, the fixation of C, as manifest in this case by experimentally induced thrombocytopenia, is directly proportional to the amount of C available for the reaction. The experiment in Fig. 7-3 demonstrates the principle that the failure to observe *in vitro* utilization of

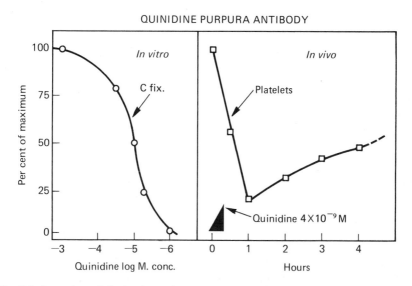

Fig. 7-3. Comparison of the *in vitro* and *in vivo* sensitivity of quinidine antibody reactions. The left graph shows the amount of complement fixed in a standard *in vitro* system containing quinidine antibody and platelets as quinidine concentration is varied. Complement fixation is the most sensitive *in vitro* test for this antibody. The right graph shows thrombocytopenia produced *in vivo* in a patient with the antibody of quinidine purpura when quinidine is infused at concen-trations too low to permit *in vitro* measurement of antibody activity. (From N. R. Shulman, *Ann. Int. Med.*, **60:**518, 1964.)

C does not exclude the participation of this system as a mediator of tissue or cell damage.

C-dependent Platelet Lysis
by Unrelated Antigen-Antibody Systems

The participation of the C system in platelet destruction by an unrelated immune event differs from the drug-induced situation. In the former instances, neither the antigen nor the antibody binds to the platelet membrane, i.e., platelet lysis does not occur unless both reactants are added to the cell suspension in the presence of fresh plasma. This reaction system therefore serves as a model for an allergic reaction which terminates in cell destruction mediated by an unrelated immune event involving C-fixing immunoglobulins. Moreover, the mechanism operative in platelet lysis probably typifies the immunopathological process described under the heading of immune complex disease discussed in Chapter 9.

Humphrey and Jaques were the first to undertake a systematic study of the allergic response of rabbit platelets about fifteen years ago. In the intervening years, considerable clarification of the phenomenon has been achieved in terms of histamine release, which, as shown below, precedes thrombocytolysis.

In this reaction system, normal rabbit platelets are suspended in a magnesium-containing buffer with fresh rabbit plasma. Upon the addition of antigen and antibody either separately or as preformed complexes in microgram quantities, the following events occur in fairly rapid succession. The platelet membranes lose their capacity to control the flow of ions as shown by an enhanced efflux of intracellular potassium, or ^{86}Rb. Shortly thereafter, histamine is released into the fluid phase as seen in Fig. 7-4, and this event is soon followed by the loss of macromolecule-associated ^{51}Cr. Platelet lysis can be observed visually or biochemically through the inability of these cells to transport ^{86}Rb from the reaction medium into the cells. This succession of responses occurs without agglutination of the platelets, and does not depend upon the presence of adenosine diphosphate in the fluid phase, although nucleotides may be released as a consequence of platelet destruction.

In contrast to the lysis of erythrocytes by antibody and C, platelet lysis does not involve prior fixation of the antibody. The impact of the immune event occurs solely through the action of immune aggregates formed in the reaction medium or added as preformed complexes in the presence of C. The specificity of the antigen is unimportant, since comparable results have been observed in experiments carried out with polysaccharide, protein, and hapten-specific immune systems. Two parameters

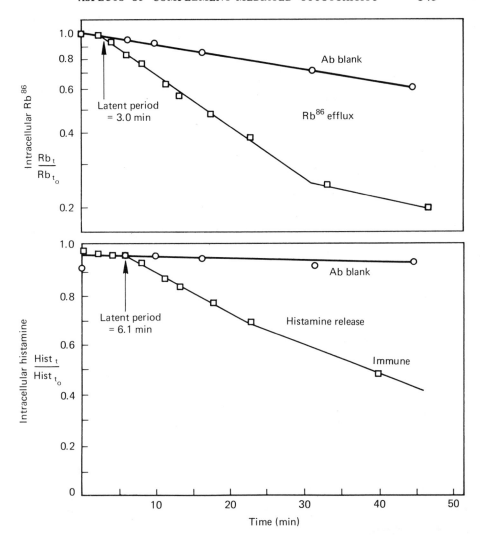

Fig. 7-4. Time course studies of the release of ^{86}Rb and histamine from rabbit platelets by an immune complex containing 4 μg of rabbit anti-ovalbumin N and 0.1 μg of antigen N in the presence of 10% normal rabbit plasma. (From A. G. Osler and R. P. Siraganian, *Prog. in Allergy,* **16:457,** 1972.)

govern the efficacy of the immune reactants with respect to the antibody. The immunoglobulins must be able to activate C, and the complexes must be formed in ratios corresponding to antibody excess or equivalence as defined by quantitative precipitation.

Opinions have differed regarding the participation of C in the allergic destruction of platelets. The major obstacles to a facile acceptance of complement's role stemmed from the observation that magnesium is by far the most important divalent cationic cofactor (calcium seems necessary at exceedingly low concentrations). Moreover, maximal effects are observed with complexes formed at antibody excess ratios rather than at the equivalence zone where C fixation in the classical manner is most effective. The uncertainty regarding the metal requirements was dissipated with the recognition that activation of the alternate pathway, a magnesium-dependent event, plays a major role in C-mediated platelet lysis. Several lines of evidence attest to the validity of this conclusion. We found that complexes containing the guinea pig gamma-1 immunoglobulins, which are inert with respect to the classical pathway but do activate the properdin system, are effective triggering agents for immunologic platelet injury. The $F(ab')_2$ dimers of the gamma-2 guinea pig antibodies whose interaction with C is also limited to the alternate pathway induce allergic platelet lysis. $F(ab')_2$ dimers prepared from rabbit antisera are similarly active as shown in Table 7-4.

Table 7–4

Allergic histamine release from rabbit platelets by various antibodies and their $F(ab')_2$ fragments

		μg antibody N per ml				
		1	2	4	8	20
Antibody		Histamine release percent				
Guinea pig antihuman serum albumin						
gamma-1	7S			65	68	44
	5S			10	35	37
gamma-2	7S			15	37	35
	5S			1	11	45
Rabbit antihuman serum albumin						
	7S	52	60	68	57	21
	5S	34		58	85	83
Rabbit antipneumococcal polysaccharide type I						
	7S	8	12	20	27	18
	5S	5	23	36	43	38

Time course studies of allergic histamine release by complexes containing the intact 7S antibody molecule or its peptic digestion product, the $F(ab')_2$ dimer, indicate that the latter is slower in onset even when the same endpoint is reached.

A summary of the factors which govern allergic platelet lysis is given in Table 7-5. These data show that platelet histamine release and lysis by

Table 7–5

Immunologic mechanisms of rabbit platelet damage by:

	Incipient immune complexes	Preformed immune aggregates
Nature of antigen	Multivalent	Multivalent
Nature of antibody	Multivalent. Fc piece is not required.	Multivalent. Fc piece is not essential.
Amount of antibody	Micrograms	Milligrams
Complement involvement	C1, C4, and C2 not essential. C3 shunt pathway required.	C6 is not needed.
Divalent cation requirements	Mg^{2+} mainly with minimal Ca^{2+}	Both Ca^{2+} and Mg^{2+}
Agglutination	May occur as a secondary manifestation.	An essential reaction step
Phagocytosis	Probably does not take place.	A crucial reaction step
Inhibitors:		
EDTA	Inhibits	Inhibits
Citrate	Inhibits	No inhibition
AMP	No inhibition	Inhibits
ADP	No effect	May enhance
Fate of platelet	Lysis follows activation of alternate pathway on membrane. Enhanced ^{86}Rb efflux precedes release of histamine and then of cytoplasmic constituents.	Phagocytosis of aggregates, activation of lysosomes, and release of cytoplasmic constituents.

C, induced by an immunologically foreign immune event, can be mediated through classical or the alternate activation pathways. However, since calcium at physiologic concentrations inhibits these events, it would follow that the alternate pathway is the main, if not the only, physiologically active mechanism. The dispensability of the Fc piece which requires calcium for C1 activity in allergic platelet lysis strengthens this conclusion. The accumulated evidence suggests that the immune complexes activate the alternate pathway in the fluid phase of the reaction medium and bind C3b. The aggregates containing this C-cleavage product adhere to the viscous platelet membrane so that the binding, assembly, and activation of the properdin enzymes lead to utilization of the late-acting C components with disruption of membrane function.

The discussion thus far has dealt with a reaction mixture containing relatively dilute platelet suspensions, $1\text{-}2 \times 10^7$ cells per ml, and immune complexes in microgram quantities. Other investigators have used more dense platelet suspensions, ca. 10^8/ml, and preformed complexes in milligram quantities. These changes incite additional mechanisms of histamine release and platelet lysis which are calcium-dependent and involve agglutination as well as the release of ADP which further intensifies agglutination and platelet destruction. Under the more concentrated conditions, phagocytosis of the immune complexes by the platelets also takes place as shown by Movat and his collaborators. This event leads to lysosomal enzyme release with further consequences to surrounding cells and tissues. A comparison between the two types of platelet damage is given in Table 7-5.

Rabbit platelets are vulnerable to still another means of immunologic attack. Immunization of rabbits, as in other species, leads to the synthesis of reaginic immunoglobulins comparable in their biologic activities to human IgE. This antibody is fixed to receptors on basophil and mast cell membranes, so that interaction of these cells with antigen leads to the release of histamine and other vasoactive substances, in a reaction considered to be C-independent. One of the compounds which is liberated from the rabbit leukocytes destroys platelets from immunized or normal rabbits. Studies of this compound have engaged the interest of several laboratories because the profound effects associated with thrombocytopenia can now be related to IgE activity. The active molecule, first shown to be released from basophils in the author's laboratory, is a small basic molecule of approximately 1000 daltons. It has been called Platelet Activating Factor (PAF), since its mode of action on platelets seemingly involves activation of a membrane enzyme related to control of intracellular adenosine $3':5'$ cyclic monophosphate. Like histamine and serotonin, PAF may function as another mediator of anaphylaxis. Current reports suggest that the human basophil may also release PAF. There are many features which distinguish this reagin- and leukocyte-dependent platelet lysis from those events initiated by immune aggregates. Some of the more important distinctions of the C-dependent allergic platelet response and the lysis which depends upon reagin-sensitized leukocytes are summarized in Table 7-6.

Studies with human platelets along the lines described above are less advanced as of this time. However experiments recently conducted by Dr. Marjorie Zucker provide highly suggestive evidence that the release of vasoactive amines, e.g., serotonin from human platelets, is also mediated by the alternate complement pathway. In these experiments, the addition of zymosan particles to human platelet-rich plasma led to the release of serotonin but without apparent platelet lysis. The reaction can be inhibited by EDTA but not by EGTA. Moreover, when the zymosan particles were removed from these reaction mixtures, washed, and added to a fresh suspension of platelets, additional release was observed. Pfueller and Lüscher subsequently supplied further evidence with regard to the role of the alternate pathway in effecting serotonin release from human platelets. They reported that the active zymosan complex which was formed on incubation with human plasma could be inhibited by cobra venom factor, hydrazine and EDTA but not by EGTA. The serotonin-releasing

Table 7–6

Allergic response of rabbit leukocytes and platelets.
Comparative reaction mechanisms.

	Rabbit platelets *	Rabbit leukocytes
1. Antibody class	IgG and others capable of activating the alternate pathway	IgE
2. Quantity required for 50% response	μg level	ng level
3. Prior fixation of antibody to cells	Nonessential; does not occur in vivo	Essential; occurs in vivo
4. Action of preformed complexes	Readily observed	Less active
5. Most efficient ratio of antibody in the complex	Antibody excess	Unknown
6. Plasma requirement	Essential	Inhibitory
7. Nature of plasma requirement	Complement-dependent	None established
8. Agglutination	Nonessential, secondary reaction	Nonessential
9. Divalent metal requirement	Magnesium	Calcium
10. Fate of cell	Cytotoxic	Probably noncytotoxic
11. Products of the reaction	Histamine, serotonin, clotting factors, and other cytoplasmic contents	Histamine plus thrombocytotoxic factor

* These parameters are applicable to platelet destruction by incipient immune complexes. Some of these characteristics may also apply to the interaction of platelets with preformed immune complexes. Compare Table 7–5.

activity of zymosan could not be reproduced with other agents known to trigger this C pathway such as inulin, bacterial lipopolysaccharides, and aggregated IgA. In agreement with previous reports, these investigators also noted that aggregated immunoglobulins could effect serotonin release in platelet-rich plasma through a mechanism involving ADP without the intervention of activated C components. While future study may reveal further differences in the responses of human and rabbit platelets, it may be anticipated that major mechanisms operative in the release of vasoactive amines from platelets of these two species are similar.

An additional effect of alternate pathway activation on platelets has been described by Zimmerman and Müller-Eberhard. These investigators found that platelet destruction by zymosan or antiplatelet antibody and C resulted in the appearance of a thrombin-like activity associated with a depletion from platelet extracts of several high molecular weight polypeptides. These alterations were observed only when intact platelets were subjected to this immunologic assault and may be related to the role of platelets in blood coagulation as discussed in Chapter 8.

FURTHER READING

Basch, R. S., "Effects of Antigen Density and Non-Complement Fixing Antibody on Cytolysis by Alloantisera," *J. Immunol.*, **113**:554, 1974.

Dacie, J. V., *The Haemolytic Anaemias,* Grune and Stratton, Inc., New York, 1967 and earlier volumes.

Ferrone, S., Cooper, N. R., Pellegrino, M. A., and Reisfeld, R. A., "The Role of Complement in the HL-A Antibody-Mediated Lysis of .Lymphocytes," *Transplantation Proc.,* **6**:13, 1974.

Fischer, J. th., Petz, L. D., Garratty, G., and Cooper, N. R., "Correlations between Quantitative Assay of Red Cell-Bound C3, Serologic Reactions, and Hemolytic Anemia," *Blood,* **44**:359, 1974.

Henson, P. M., and Cochrane, C. G., "Acute Immune Complex Disease in Rabbits. The Role of Complement and of a Leukocyte-Dependent Release of Vasoactive Amines from Platelets," *J. Exp. Med.,* **133**:554, 1971, and earlier papers.

Marney, S. R., Colley, D. G., and Des Prez, R. M., "Alternate Complement Pathway Induction of Aggregation and Release of S-Hydroxytryptamine and Adenosine Diphosphate by Rabbit Platelets," *J. Immunol.,* **114**:696, 1975.

Osler, A. G., and Siraganian, R. P., "Immunologic Mechanisms of Platelet Damage," *Prog. in Allergy,* **16**:450, 1972.

Pellegrino, M. A., Ferrone, S., Cooper, N. R., Dierich, M. P., and Reisfeld, R. A., "Variation in Susceptibility of a Human Lymphoid Cell Line to Immune Lysis During the Cell Cycle," *J. Exp. Med.,* **140**:578, 1974.

Perlmann, P., Perlmann, H., and Lachmann, P., "Lymphocyte-Associated Complement: Role of C8 in Certain Cell-mediated Lytic Reactions, *Scan. Jour. Immunology,* **3**:77, 1974.

Rosse, W. F., "Quantitative Immunology of Immune Hemolytic Anemia," *J. Clin. Invest.,* **50**:727, 734, 1971.

Shulman, N. R., "A Mechanism of Cell Destruction in Individuals Sensitized to Foreign Antigens and Its Implications in Auto-immunity," *Ann. Internal Med.,* **60**:506, 1964.

Winn, H. J., Baldamus, C. A., Jooste, S. V., and Russell, P. S., "Acute Destruction by Humoral Antibody of Rat Skin Grafted to Mice. The Role of Complement and Polymorphonuclear Leukocytes," *J. Exp. Med.,* **137**:893, 1973.

Chapter 8

Complement and Inflammation

Although the title of this chapter might have been considered unduly speculative some fifteen years ago, the participation of C in inflammatory reactions is now one of the dominant themes in this research area. Justification for this statement stems from the realization that events such as the release of histamine and kinins, contraction of smooth muscle, separation of contiguous endothelial cells of the vascular system resulting in enhanced permeability, leukotaxis, lysosomal enzyme release, and initiation of blood coagulation all have been demonstrated to follow activation of the C system. Several of these events are dependent upon the properties of the anaphylatoxins which are discussed below.

ANAPHYLATOXINS: FORMATION AND CHARACTERIZATION

The term "anaphylatoxin" was originally applied to a fluid-phase property of "activated" serum which, on injection into normal guinea pigs, reproduced a clinical picture resembling systemic anaphylaxis. Since "activation" of the serum was achieved by such unrelated substances as agar, inulin, denatured proteins, various microorganisms as well as by antigen-antibody complexes, this process was not generally considered to be immunologic in nature. In 1959, studies in our laboratory showed that utilization of the late-acting C components resulted in anaphylatoxin production, a conclusion based on the following experimental results:

Incubation of an immune aggregate with fresh but not with heated rat serum at 37° C led to a loss of overall hemolytic activity and consumption of the late components. A diminution in this C function was accompanied by a concurrent increase in the ability of the treated serum to contract the guinea pig ileum and enhance vascular permeability. These tissue effects were more pronounced when the serum was pretreated with immune aggregates formed at equivalence rather than at antigen excess ratios, in accordance with the results of C-fixation assays.

149

Although a loss of hemolytic C activity also occurred after incubation of these reaction mixtures for 18 hr at 0° C, late component activity was not diminished. Neither were the biologic manifestations observed. The latter two effects were highly temperature-dependent.

The admixture of agar or high molecular weight dextrans with serum at 37° C produced results similar to those of immune aggregates, i.e., consumption of C activity accompanied by anaphylatoxin production. The degree of smooth muscle contraction and permeability enhancement by the supernates of C-fixation reaction mixtures was proportional to the loss in the hemolytic activity of the late-acting components, collectively called C3 at that time. Moreover, hydrazine and phlorizin, inhibitors of C3 activity, also suppressed the production of anaphylatoxic properties in C-fixation reaction mixtures. These findings established the immunologic nature of anaphylatoxin as a consequence of C activation.

Since the publication of these findings, the work of several investigators has led to the isolation of the active products and to confirmation of their relationships to the C system. In 1967 Lepow, Dias da Silva, and their associates established that the anaphylatoxic activity in human serum could be attributed to a minor cleavage product of C3, now called C3a, and postulated a molecular weight of 9000 for this fragment. They also succeeded in generating anaphylatoxic activity through the addition of purified $\overline{C1}$, C4, C2, and magnesium to human serum. Comparative studies of human and rat serum anaphylatoxins showed that the human C3a did not desensitize the guinea pig ileum to contraction by the anaphylatoxin produced in rat serum by agar. The basis for this difference was clarified by Jensen, who found that cleavage of C5 in guinea pig serum also generated a product with anaphylatoxic activity. Similar results were achieved through the interaction of purified C components and immune complexes or, more simply, by subjecting purified C5 to tryptic digestion. It thus became apparent that there were two anaphylatoxins, one formed through cleavage of C3 and the other, C5a, by fragmentation of C5.

Studies of human C3a and C5a in Müller-Eberhard's laboratory have shown that these peptides are cleaved from the N-terminal portion of C3 and C5; they have been assigned the properties listed in Table 8-1.

For a number of years, the human C3a and C5a peptides were not considered functional because of the inability to generate biological activity in human serum. This erroneous conclusion has now been corrected by the demonstration of a highly active anaphylatoxin inhibitor in human serum. This inhibitor has been identified as the carboxypeptidase B-like enzyme described by Erdös which removes the C-terminal arginine with a concomitant loss of biological activity. The incorporation of an inhibitor of carboxypeptidase B, epsilon-aminocaproic acid, has permitted the isolation of active C3a and C5a from human serum. This enzyme inhibitor is

Table 8–1

Properties of human anaphylatoxins *

	Human C3a	Human C5a
Molecular weight	9000	17,000
Electrophoretic mobility at pH = 8.5 $\times$ 10^{-5} cm^2 V^{-1} sec^{-1}	+2.1	−1.7
N-terminal amino acid	Serine	
C-terminal amino acid	Arginine	Probably arginine
Formation by classical pathway enzyme	C$\overline{42}$	C$\overline{423}$
Formation by alternate pathway enzyme	C3 Activator ($\overline{B}$)	Serum activation by inulin
Threshold quantity for contraction of smooth muscle	1.1×10^{-8} M	7.5×10^{-10} M
Threshold quantity for wheal and erythema in human skin	2×10^{-12} mol	1×10^{-15} mol
Formation by action of noncomplement enzymes on purified component	Trypsin and plasmin	Trypsin and plasmin

* Based largely on data from Vallota, E. H., and Müller-Eberhard, H. J., J. Exp. Med., 137:1109, 1973.

either lacking or of feeble potency in pig, rat, and guinea pig sera since anaphylatoxic peptides can be readily generated in these sera by the addition of zymosan, inulin, or immune aggregates, in the absence of epsilon-aminocaproate. Insofar as they have been characterized, both C3a and C5a derived from human or porcine sera contain a basic amino acid as the carboxy terminal residue which is essential for smooth muscle contraction.

Hugli, Morgan, Vallota, and Müller-Eberhard demonstrated that both C3a and C5a have considerable helical structure, with nearly identical spectra in the far-ultraviolet region. Treatment with reducing agents reversibly diminishes both the conformation and biological activity of these peptides. These findings indicate that the presence of the carboxy terminal arginine and the integrity of the secondary structure of the molecule are required for interaction with the leukocyte membrane for full expression of anaphylatoxic activity. Hugli et al have recently established the amino acid composition and partial sequence of C3a and C5a. Numerous differences are evident. C3a is very acid-stable. It contains no tryptophane residues and two sequences of Cys·Cys. The C5a molecule has a much higher ratio of tyrosine to phenylalanine than does C3a. The potency of these mediators of inflammation can be readily appreciated by the finding that they are ten times more active than bradykinin.

The participation of the alternate pathway in anaphylatoxin production was readily demonstrated by incubating guinea pig gamma-1 immune complexes with guinea pig or rat serum. Similarly, endotoxin, which consumes the late-acting components (C3–C9) with but scanty utilization of C1, C4, or C2, also produces anaphylatoxins. Preliminary reports suggest that the C4a fragments may constitute a third anaphylatoxic peptide, but little information is as yet available concerning this complement-derived product.

BIOLOGIC PROPERTIES OF ANAPHYLATOXINS

Histamine Release

A salient feature of anaphylatoxin activity is the capacity to release vasoactive compounds such as histamine and serotonin from tissue mast cells and blood basophils. This process, which has been visualized by Pondman and his colleagues, results in local wheal and erythema formation in the mammalian skin and is accompanied by degranulation of the mast cell cytoplasmic granules containing these pharmacologically active agents. Extensive studies on the mechanism of amine release have been conducted with the polyamine 48/80 by Uvnäs or with the action of antigen on sensitized tissue mast cells or blood basophils. It is not clear at this writing whether the anaphylatoxins act in a similar manner. However, Dr. Alice Johnson has demonstrated that antigen-induced histamine release differs mechanistically from that mediated by 48/80. Some of the differences are summarized in Table 8-2. It is interesting to note that antirat gamma globulin (anti-RGG) which releases histamine through a cytotoxic C-dependent mechanism differs in several respects from the mode of histamine release mediated by antigen or 48/80. With respect to the latter, Uvnäs proposes that histamine is displaced from the cytoplasmic granules by cation exchange, presumably without cell death.

Table 8–2

Release of substances from rat mast cells *

Substance	Intracellular location	Releasing agent †			
		48/80	Antigen	Anti-RGG	Other
LDH	cytoplasm	−	−	−	+
ATP	cytoplasm				
	mitochondria	−	−	−	+
Serotonin	granules	+	+	0	+
Histamine	granules	+	+	+	+
Potassium	cytoplasm	−	−	0	+
	granules	+	+	0	+

* Modified from Johnson, A. R., and Moran, N. C., *Cellular and Humoral Mechanisms in Anaphylaxis and Allergy*, H. Z. Movat, Ed., S. Karger, Basel, 1969, p. 122.

† Symbol + means released and − means not released. Symbol 0 means not determined. "Other agents" refers to surface active compounds such as Triton X-100 or n-decylamine.

Smooth Muscle Contraction

The ability of C3a and C5a to contract smooth muscle represents one of the early demonstrations of anaphylatoxin activities. Repeated application of the same peptide results in tachyphylaxis, i.e., a temporary diminution in muscle contractility. These tissues evidently possess different receptors for C3a and C5a, since the two anaphylatoxins do not induce cross-tachyphylaxis. Wissler has recently claimed that the enhancement of capillary permeability by the anaphylatoxins is due to a different compound than that which induces smooth muscle contraction, but these reports have not yet been confirmed in other laboratories. Both manifestations of these C-derived peptides may in fact be due to the same process. Majno has offered a convincing demonstration that the edema produced by histamine or serotonin, which can be released by the anaphylatoxins, is due to a shortening of the contractile elements in the endothelial cells lining the post-capillary venules, which results in the separation of contiguous endothelial cells. A graphic representation of this process, taken from the studies of Majno and Palade, is reproduced in Fig. 8-1.

Leukotaxis

Interest in the C system as a mediator of tissue damage received further impetus through the discovery that anaphylatoxins as well as the high molecular weight $\overline{C567}$ complex promote leukotaxis, the directed migration of leukocytes across a concentration gradient. Virtually all types of white blood cells are susceptible to this influence which has been attributed by Becker to the activation of one or more cell-bound serine esterases.

The data in Fig. 8-2 demonstrate an important *in vivo* consequence of C activation attributable to a low molecular weight molecule, possibly anaphylatoxin. McCall and his colleagues found that intravenous injection of cobra venom factor or inulin into rabbits resulted in an immediate and severe neutropenia. As shown in Fig. 8-2, peripheral levels of polymorphonuclear cells fell dramatically within minutes after the administration of these activators of the alternate or properdin pathway. These authors tentatively suggest that the neutropenia is due to sequestration rather than lysis of the cells. In either event, the diminished cell count is followed within two hours or so by a marked neutrophilia, reaching levels which are 5 times above normal. It is tempting to speculate that the leukopenia may somehow be related to the depression of antibody synthesis following cobra factor treatment of animals, as discussed in Chapter 6. Further, is the leukocytosis, first described by Rother as the leukocyte-mobilizing phenomenon, due to the chemotactic property of the anaphylatoxins?

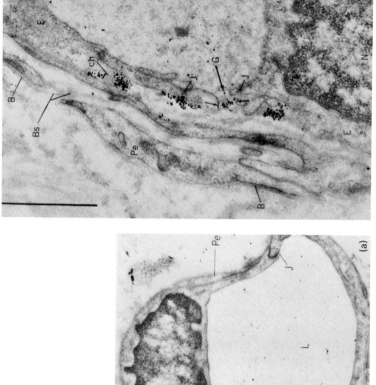

Fig. 8-1. Abbreviations: B, basement membrane; G, gap in the endothelium; J, intercellular junction; N, nucleus; E, endothelial cell. (a) A capillary, 4 min after the local injection of serotonin and intravenous injection of colloidal HgS. There is no evidence of injury. Particles of HgS are visible in the lumen; none are present in the vascular wall. Magnification: 16,000. (b) Part of a leaking vessel 4 min after the injection of serotonin and intravenous injection of HgS. Example of an endothelial gap at an early stage. Tracer particles are present between the margins of the gap (G), while other particles have penetrated between the layers of the wall. Magnification: 45,000. (From G. Majno, and G. E. Palade, J. Biophys. and Biochem. Cytol., 11:571, 1961.)

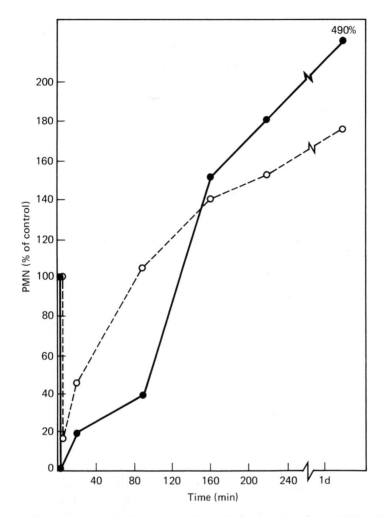

Fig. 8-2. Effects of intravenous administration of 1.0 ml of cobra venon factor (●) or 50 mg of inulin (○) on rabbit peripheral blood PMN counts. Values are expressed as percentages of control value, which was obtained 1–5 min before infection. The values are representative experiments, selected from more than five individual observations, all done in duplicate. (From C. E. McCall, L. R. De Chatelet, D. Brown, and P. Lachmann, *Nature*, **249**:841, 1974.)

Neutrophils   C-derived chemotactic factors for neutrophils are three in number: C3a, C5a, and the intermediate complex containing C567. As noted previously, the cleavage products of C3 and C5 can be produced through the action of enzymes formed during the sequence of component activation or by enzymes which are extrinsic to the C system. The latter include trypsin, plasmin, thrombin, as well as certain tissue and bacterial proteases which can utilize C3 and C5 as substrates but do not sustain sequential component interactions. Possibly enzymes with similar substrate specificities will be found to explain the chemotactic activity of diverse biological materials. One which is of interest because it links the kinin-generating and C systems is the kininogenase in human serum. Antigen-stimulated lymphoid cells have also been found to secrete a chemotactic factor for neutrophils.

Since C3a and C5a represent products of C activation through the classical or alternate pathways, it was anticipated that immune activation would induce chemotactic activity. This was shown to be the case for neu-trophil chemotaxis (Table 8-3). Normal guinea pig serum activated by homologous gamma-1 immunoglobulins generated chemotactic activity for neutrophils, as did serum from C4-deficient guinea pigs. The activity pro-duced by either gamma-1 or gamma-2 antibodies was apparently due to C5a since it was nullified by the addition of an antiserum to C5 but not by anti-C3.

As noted above, Rother has described a C-dependent leukocyte-mobi-

Table 8–3

Effect of rabbit anti-C3 and anti-C5 on chemotactic activity generated by preformed complexes of γ1 or γ2 immunoglobulins in guinea pig serum *

	Chemotactic activity ‡	
Preparation †	1	2
Supernatant of guinea pig serum incubated with:		
γ1 immune complex		
plus buffer	252	274
plus normal rabbit serum	202	nt §
plus anti-C3	252	216
plus anti-C5	29	46
γ2 immune complex		
plus buffer	214	240
plus normal rabbit serum	206	nt
plus anti-C3	204	216
plus anti-C5	38	22

* From Sandberg, A. L., Snyderman, R., Frank, M. M., and Osler, A. G., J. Immunol., 108:1230, 1972.

† The supernates of normal guinea pig serum incubated with γ1 or γ2 guinea pig preformed immune aggregates (PIA) for 60 min at 37°C were filtered through a column of Sephadex G-100. Portions (0.8 ml) of the peaks of chemotactic activity were incubated for 30 min at 37°C with 0.025 ml of inactivated (56°C, 30 min) normal rabbit serum or rabbit anti-guinea pig C3 or C5. The reaction mixtures were brought to 1.7 ml with Gey's medium and tested for chemotac-tic activity.

‡ Expressed as cells per high power field in five experiments performed in duplicate.

§ nt, not tested.

lizing factor produced by the interaction of C1, C4, and C2 with C3 which seems to differ from C3a. The activity, assayed in terms of white-cell mobilization under *in vitro* or *in vivo* conditions has been detected with human, rabbit, guinea pig, rat, and mouse sera. Within four minutes after injection of the activated sera into rabbits, the peripheral white count rose from 4×10^3 to 9×10^3 leukocytes per mm^3. A molecular weight in the range of 7000 to 12,000 daltons has been assigned to this factor. Smith and his colleagues have reported that $\overline{C1}$INH enhances leukotaxis in addition to having an inhibitory action on $\overline{C1}$.

Eosinophils   Attention has been directed to these cells in view of their close association with allergic disorders. Kay has reported that eosinophils respond to C5a generated in guinea pig serum by gamma-1 or gamma-2 immunoglobulins. As in the case for neutrophils, a number of chemotatic factors have been described. The degree of heterogeneity is indicated by the fact that several are unrelated to C activation and the assignment of molecular weights which range from less than 1000 to 15,000. With but one exception, few of these factors are specific for a single cell type. It is therefore apparent that the directed migration of leukocytes can be induced by a variety of stimuli capable of cell membrane perturbation or activation of membrane-bound serine esterases as postulated by Becker. This suggestion receives considerable support from Majno's findings to the effect that the contractile elements in blood leukocytes may be involved in the cells' mobility and that their function is enzyme-regulated.

Human basophils also exhibit relatively weak chemotaxis in the presence of C5a, C567, plasma kallikrein, and supernates from sensitized lymphocytes incubated with specific antigen.

Mononuclear cells   The chemotactic effect of C3a and C5a for mononuclear cells has led some observers to suggest that the C system participates in some aspects of cell-mediated immune phenomena. As with the other leukocytes, there seems to be no selectivity in the sense that the migration of certain cell types is promoted by specific factors. This statement applies to the tissue and bacterial proteases as well as the C-derived anaphylatoxins.

Lymphocytes have been reported to respond to culture fluids obtained from antigen-stimulated sensitized cells, a process which may account for the presence of relatively large numbers of unsensitized lymphocytes at the sites of delayed hypersensitivity reactions.

Release of Lysosomal Enzymes

An additional property has recently been assigned to one of the human anaphylatoxins, 5a. Evidence obtained in the author's laboratory, in collaboration with Drs. Goldstein and Weissmann, led to the conclusion that this peptide mediates the release of lysosomal enzymes from human polymorphonuclear leukocytes pretreated with cytochalasin B. Fresh human sera treated with zymosan, specific immune complexes, or cobra venom factor and centrifuged at high speed were found to induce the release of β-glucuronidase and myeloperoxidase, but not of cytoplasmic enzymes like lactic dehydrogenase from autologous leukocytes. Enzyme release was not apparent unless the cells had been exposed to cytochalasin B at a concentration of 5 μg per ml. Although the mechanism of this release process has not yet been clarified, it appears that a process of "reverse endocytosis" may be at work. This mechanism seemingly involves contact of C5a with the cell's plasma membrane, leading to a fusion of the granules with the membrane and lysosomal enzyme release. Electron micrographs show a merger of the granule and cell membranes and a reduction in the number of lysosomes in the cytoplasm. An increased activity of the hexose monophosphate shunt of leukocytes has been associated with this process. In addition, the lysosomal enzymes include a protease which may increase the available C5a through its cleavage of C5. The activity of the lysosomal lysates may also involve enzymatic conversion of Factor B to $\overline{\text{B}}$. In these studies the C5a anaphylatoxin was generated through the alternate pathway with the use of selective activators as noted above. Moreover C5a formation and lysosomal enzyme release was inhibited by EDTA and salicylaldoxime but not by EGTA. The active product was characterized as a molecule of 15,000 to 20,000 molecular weight which was chemotactic for polymorphonuclear cells and was identified as a C5a fragment with the aid of specific antisera. Purified human C5 treated with trypsin yielded a product with similar properties.

Treatment of fresh, but not heated, human serum with graded amounts of zymosan lowered the C3PA activity of the serum to an extent that was inversely proportional to the supernate's lysosomal enzyme-releasing potency as shown in Table 8-4.

Neutrophilic leukocytes are not the only cells whose lysosomal enzymes can cleave C5 with the production of chemotactic factors. Proteases derived from macrophage or platelet lysosomes yield similar fragments linking these cells to inflammation and blood coagulation.

The consequences of C activation which involve leukotaxis and lysosomal enzyme release underscore the role of this system as a mediator of inflammation.

OTHER PERMEABILITY FACTORS

In addition to C3a and C5a, other byproducts of C interaction have been described which act as kinins and increase vascular permeability. One of these is thought to be the 9000–11,000 fragment, C4a, cleaved from C4

Table 8–4

Cobra venom factor activation of the alternate pathway and
enzyme releasing activity in zymosan treated serum * (ZTS) †

	CVFAH$_{50}$ ‡	B-Glucuronidase released §
	units/ml	%
Fresh serum	31.1	8.4
ZTS (0.1 mg/ml)	26.9	9.3
ZTS (0.5 mg/ml)	16.5	11.7
ZTS (1.0 mg/ml)	9.5	14.0

* Serum incubated with zymosan at 37°C for 15 min before filtration. PMNs preincubated 15 min with 5 µg/ml cytochalasin B.

† From Goldstein, I. M., Brai, M., Osler, A. G., and Weissmann, G., J. Immunol., 111:33, 1973.

‡ Cobra venom factor activable hemolysis of unsensitized erythrocytes, i.e., C3PA activity units.

§ Expressed as percent of total activity released into supernatant by 0.2% Triton X-100 (13.5 ± 0.82 µg phenolphthalein/2 × 10^{6}PMN.

by C$\overline{1}$s at pH = 7.4. Its presence is demonstrable by its capacity to contract the isolated rat uterus.

A C2-dependent permeability factor has been described which is demonstrable in man. Its action is not inhibitable by antihistamines. A requirement for C2 but not C3 in the formation of this agent indicates that this factor is not C3a. Although this permeability factor has not been well characterized, it is thought to play a major role in the edema associated with hereditary angioedema, described previously as a disorder associated with diminished C$\overline{1}$INH activity in the sera of affected patients. Donaldson has shown that sera from nonsymptomatic patients will generate this permeability factor in the presence of C4 and C2. Antisera to these components will prevent its generation. Antibody to C3 is without effect. This permeability-enhancing agent has been distinguished from C4a and bradykinin in terms of amino acid composition and its inactivation by trypsin and chymotrypsin.

BLOOD COAGULATION

The findings of Ratnoff and Lepow concerning the activation of C$\overline{1}$ by plasmin and the demonstration by Donaldson that kallikrein can activate C$\overline{1}$ *in vitro* opened new avenues of investigation which revealed important interrelationships between the C system, kinin formation, and blood coagulation. Briefly stated, activation of the Hageman factor and its fragmentation leads to conversion of plasma prekallikrein to kallikrein which converts C1 to its catalytic, esteratic forms. The conversion of C1 to C$\overline{1}$ is also mediated by plasmin, which is derived from plasminogen by activated

Hageman factor. Thus activated Hageman factor leads to $C\overline{1}$ formation via plasmin and kallikrein, the latter being responsible for the cleavage of bradykinin from its kininogen. The pertinence of these relationships to the C system is further emphasized by the finding in Austen's laboratory to the effect that $C\overline{1}INH$ inhibits not only $C\overline{1}$, but also blood coagulation, fibrinolysis, and kinin generation. The major steps in this sequence which is currently under active investigation are traced in Fig. 8-3. A note of caution regarding the ability of enzymes in the blood coagulation to inactivate C components is suggested in a recent report by Campbell and Nelson. These investigators found that highly purified thrombin, in contrast to the commercially available preparations, was devoid of activity in the C system.

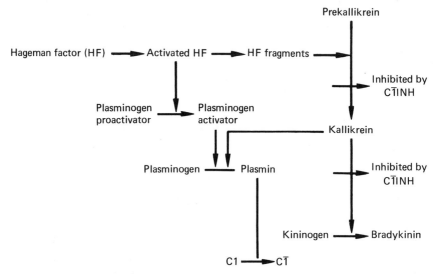

Fig. 8-3. (Modified from K. F. Austen, *Transplantation Proc.*, 6:40, 1974.)

Complement involvement in blood coagulation relates to the activation of the $C\overline{1}$ esterase not only by Hageman factor as just mentioned, but by other means as well. Initial evidence was provided by Robbins and Stetson, who showed that the interaction of antigen with antibody in whole rabbit blood accelerated clot formation. The relationship of this finding to the C system was established when it was observed that blood clotting time was prolonged and prothrombin consumption delayed in the blood of C6-deficient rabbits. In normal rabbit blood, coagulation was associated with minor decrements of C6 and C7. Although a direct relationship between C and blood clotting was initially postulated, it has been shown that the coagulation defect in rabbits lacking C6 stemmed from the inability of C6-deficient plasma to promote allergic platelet lysis. Destruction of the platelets with the release of blood coagulation factors accounted for the observations of Robbins and Stetson. The prolongation of blood clotting in C6-deficient rabbits could be corrected by adding C6, one of the terminal components essential for thrombocytolysis. Platelet lysis via the C system results in the loss of high molecular weight polypeptides from the platelets in a manner similar to platelet destruction by thrombin.

FURTHER READING

Becker, E. L., "The Relation of Enzyme Activation to Mediator Secretion and Chemotactic Response," in *Mechanisms in Allergy*, Goodfriend, Sehon, and Orange, Eds., Marcel Dekker, Inc., New York, 1973, p. 339.

Donaldson, V. H., "Blood Coagulation and Related Plasma Enzymes in Inflammation," *Ser. Haemat.*, 3:39, 1970.

Goldstein, I. M., Brai, M., Osler, A. G., and Weissmann, G., "Lysosomal Enzyme Release from Human Leukocytes: Mediation by the Alternate Pathway of Complement Activation," *J. Immunol.*, 111:33, 1973.

Hugli, T. E., Vallota, E. H., and Müller-Eberhard, H. J., "Purification and Partial Characterization of Human and Porcine C3a Anaphylatoxin," *J. Biol. Chem.*, 250:1472, 1975.

Johnson, A. R., Hugli, T. E., and Müller-Eberhard, H. J., "Release of Histamine from Rat Mast Cells by the Complement Peptides C3a and C5a," *Immunology*, 28:1067, 1975.

Lepow, I. H., Dias da Silva, W., and Patrick, R. A. in *Cellular and Humoral Mechanisms in Anaphylaxis and Allergy*, Austen and Becker, Eds., Karger, Basel, 1966, p. 237.

Müller-Eberhard, H. J., Vallota, E. H., Götze, O., and Zimmerman, T. S., *Mediators of the Inflammatory Response—Complement in Inflammation*, I. H. Lepow and P. A. Ward, Eds. Academic Press, New York, 1972, p. 83.

Osler, A. G., Randall, H. G., Hill, B. M., and Ovary, Z., "The Participation of Complement in the Formation of Anaphylatoxin," *J. Exp. Med.*, 110:311, 1959.

Vallota, E. H., and Müller-Eberhard, H. J., "Formation of C3a and C5a Anaphylatoxins in Whole Human Serum After Inhibition of the Anaphylatoxin Inactivator," *J. Exp. Med.*, 137:1109, 1973.

Ward, P. A., "Complement-Derived Leukotactic Factors in Pathological Fluids," *J. Exp. Med.*, 134:No. 3, Part 2, p. 109s, 1971.

Chapter 9

Other Types of

Complement-associated Tissue Injury

The advances achieved in our understanding of the mechanisms of C action at the biochemical and molecular levels have been accompanied by extensive efforts to evaluate the role of C in a wide array of immunopathological events. Many of the investigations have been restricted to the demonstration of an association between changes in serum C or component levels with the type of tissue injury under study. The significance of these correlative studies has often been difficult to evaluate. Now that highly purified reagents are available and a more precise understanding of several of the component interaction mechanisms is at hand, it would seem appropriate to review the criteria whose fulfillment could establish a causative role for C in tissue damage.

The type of evidence required to distinguish a causal from a casual relationship between C activation and tissue damage will necessarily vary with the nature and complexity of the latter. In some instances unequivocal conclusions are more easily attainable. Thus there can be little doubt regarding the phlogistic attributes of the anaphylatoxins when the intradermal injection of a few nanograms of highly purified and well-characterized C3a or C5a produces an immediate wheal and flare reaction in the skin with concomitant degranulation of the mast cells. The development of *in vitro* models which reproduce all aspects of these tissue-damaging events provides thoroughly convincing proof. In more complex situations, rigorous evidence of this nature is more difficult to assemble. The tell-tale clues of tissue deposits of immune complexes and of C components are suggestive of C-mediated tissue damage. However, evidence furnished by such findings may not be conclusive. The immune complexes associated with the lesion site may not contain C-activating immunoglobulins. Non-C-derived enzymes of bacterial origin can also account for the cleavage of various C components including C3 and C5. Lysosomal enzymes liberated from leukocytes or platelets, destroyed by C-independent mechanisms, can also contribute to the immunopathologic events. Although such findings do not deny a biologic role for the anaphylatoxins, they cannot be taken to indicate a primary pathogenetic role for antigen-antibody aggregates. Further examples include the clustering of C4 and the deposition of C3b at sites removed from the progressing lesion. Proteins from staphylococci and streptococci can activate the C system thereby inflicting tissue injury of a secondary nature. Similar considerations apply to the C-reactive protein.

Abrogation of the tissue response in animals depleted of one or more C components through hereditary or experimental means constitutes significant evidence for the putative role of C, particularly if the tissue lesion can be restored with purified, monofunctional components. Finally the construction of theoretically valid *in vitro* models can be of great utility in resolving the issue of C-dependence. These and other approaches have found a prominent place in C research. Their contributions and limitations are evaluated below.

C IN ANAPHYLAXIS MEDIATED BY IMMUNOGLOBULINS OTHER THAN IgE

Passive cutaneous anaphylaxis (PCA), as extensively developed by Ovary, is the most widely used model in this regard. This allergic response is induced as follows. Varying concentrations of antibody are injected intradermally and followed within several hours by the intravenous inoculation of the antigen admixed with a dye such as Evans Blue. The immune event at the site of antibody deposition leads to an extravasation of plasma proteins. In view of the firm binding of the dye to albumin, skin-blueing is visualized within minutes. The area of blueing is proportional to the intensity of the antigen-antibody reaction, provided several criteria have been fulfilled. These include the use of multivalent antigen and a bivalent immunoglobulin whose Fc piece is intact and capable of relatively firm binding to an appropriate tissue site. The interaction of the antigen with the cell-bound immunoglobulin in guinea pig skin leads to fusion of the histamine-containing vesicle membranes with the plasma membrane of the mast cell and extrusion of vasoactive amines. The action of histamine, like that of serotonin and bradykinin, has been described by Majno and collaborators. They have proposed the following sequence to account for the cutaneous edema which is visualized grossly by skin blueing. The reactions include dilatation of the post-venule capillaries, leading to increased pressure in these blood vessels and in the venules, and also contraction and separation of the endothelial cells with development of leaks. Contraction of the endothelial cells is considered as the response which underlies the two major effects of these mediators, e.g., stimulation of smooth muscle and enhanced vascular permeability. Histamine liberators such as C3a and C5a act through these means.

Evidence in accord with the participation of the C system as an effector of this response was obtained from studies in our laboratory with a model of PCA in the rat induced by rabbit and horse antibodies. In these studies, a close correlation was observed between the extent of skin-blueing in the rat and the degree of C fixation by these heterologous immune systems. Moreover, dose-response experiments indicated that the extent of skin-blueing could be modulated by quantitative changes in the *in vivo* availability of hemolytic C. Thus when 12 μg of antibody N was injected intradermally and the animals challenged several hours later with 12 μg of homologous antigen, the diameters of the cutaneous reactions were:

1. In normal rats   13 mm
2. In normal rats injected with fresh guinea pig or
   rat serum   22 mm
3. In C-depleted rats   2 mm
4. In C-depleted rats injected with fresh rat serum   11 mm

This correlation was extended in the demonstration that restoration of the skin-blueing was quantitatively dependent on the available quantity of the late C components, called C′3 in 1957. For example, the intravenous injection of as little as 2.5 mg of zymosan per rat completely abolished the animal's capacity to support passive cutaneous anaphylaxis. In retrospect, this and other findings suggest that depletion of alternate pathway components was possibly associated with anaphylactic unresponsiveness. We have also observed that phlorizin, an inhibitor of the C system at the $\overline{EAC142}$ stage, also suppressed local and systemic anaphylaxis in the guinea pig. When guinea pigs were passively sensitized with 50 μg of rabbit antibody N and challenged twenty hours later with 5 μg of antigen N, anaphylactic death occurred in about 75% of the animals. An injection of phlorizin one hour prior to challenge with antigen protected the majority of the guinea pigs (ca. 70%) from a fatal reaction. In the light of subsequent findings by other investigators, a qualifying consideration must be entered. Under *in vitro* conditions, it has not been possible to demonstrate firm fixation of the immunoglobulins which induce the anaphylactic reactions to rat mast cells. It is therefore plausible to interpret the skin reactions as due, in part at least, to the action of rat serum anaphylatoxins which were generated at the cutaneous site of the antibody-antigen reaction. In these circumstances, the mechanism of histamine or serotonin liberation therefore differs from that of the cutaneous wheal and erythema response promoted by reaginic antibodies of the IgE class. A similar interpretation may be applicable to the findings by Austen and collaborators, who also concluded that PCA in the rat mediated by a subclass of homologous IgG immunoglobulins is C-dependent. Additional evidence of an indirect and correlative nature has been provided by Ovary and his collaborators. They showed that guinea pig IgG1, whose activation of the C system is limited to the alternate pathway, is a potent effector of PCA reactions in the homologous species.

The implications of these findings with respect to C involvement have been countered by other observations. Thus reduction of C3 levels in the guinea pig to less than 10% of their normal values by the injection of the cobra venom factor failed to reduce the intensity of PCA responses. Moreover, C4-deficient guinea pigs also support PCA reactions. Some resolution of these controversial findings may be referable to the use of guinea pigs as the test animal and to the class of immunoglobulin selected for the skin sensitization. Casey and Tokuda differentiated several types of PCA reactions in the mouse with respect to the sensitizing antibody, duration of the latent period, and C-dependency. A putative role for the C system in the mediation of this anaphylactic response was indicated when rabbit but not mouse IgG antibodies were used with a latent period of one hour. The possible implication of C-dependent platelet lysis in the development of skin-blueing at the local sensitization site must also be considered in evaluating the mechanism of these reactions. Clearly, the available data do not yet permit a definitive interpretation regarding the role of C in PCA reactions mediated by immunoglobulins of the IgG class.

ALLERGIC REACTIONS MEDIATED BY IgE

The construction of a relatively simple *in vitro* system for the study of IgE-mediated histamine release facilitated the accumulation of evidence which seems to exclude a role for C in these allergic reactions. Briefly summarized, we have shown that human leukocytes suspended in a buffer solution lacking an exogenous supply of serum could be deprived of virtually all their C1, C4, and C2 and still release histamine on interaction with antigen, fully as well as untreated cells from the same donor. Moreover, the release of histamine could be abruptly and irreversibly interrupted by the addition of chelating agents such as ethylenediaminetetraacetate at any stage of the process. In view of these findings, we concluded that the allergic release of histamine represents an enhanced secretory response without cytolysis. This conclusion has been confirmed by Hastie on the basis of morphological studies. Lichtenstein and Margolis extended this conclusion in the important demonstration that the allergic release of this amine is governed by the intracellular level of cyclic adenosine monophosphate, cAMP. These significant observations were supplemented by the work of May and his collaborators, who observed that the allergenic release of histamine was not accompanied by the concurrent loss of the lysosomal enzyme, beta-glucuronidase. In contrast, the phagocytosis of zymosan particles, a C-dependent process, led to the release of this enzyme but not of histamine. Although modulation of intracellular cAMP as a regulator of immune histamine release is generally conceived to be independent of the C system, the recent report of Kaline and Austen is of interest in this regard. They noted that pharmacologic inhibition of cAMP breakdown in rat mast cells, a step associated with histamine release, also suppressed C-mediated cytolysis. The later finding that aggregated IgE activated the alternate but not the classical C pathway in a rather feeble manner raised some doubts about C involvement, but these were soon dispelled when Grant and Lichtenstein found that the content of C3 in the fluid phase of reaction mixtures or on the leukocyte membranes exerted no influence on immune histamine liberation by IgE. Extrapolation of these *in vitro* findings to the wheal and flare reactions caused by IgE bound to mast cells in the human skin seems well justified, but several mitigating considerations still require discussion. The release of histamine in the test tube can be activated by picogram quantities of antigen so that perturbations of the C system, if they did occur, would be undetectable by currently available methods. Further, as indicated in Chapter 4, activation of the classical C system by an immune aggregate varies directly with the amount of C in the reaction system. It is therefore conceivable, albeit unlikely, that the degree of C activation which may occur *in vivo* represents but a minute fraction of the available supply and therefore escapes detection. Furthermore, the formation of anaphylatoxins or the deposition of alternate pathway components on the mast cell membrane in amounts sufficient to cause degranulation has not been excluded. The fact that heated human serum contains dialyzable materials capable of enhancing the *in vitro* response is consistent with the properties of C3a and C5a, but the action of substances other than anaphylatoxins can also be invoked to explain these findings. Moreover, the role of alternate pathway components in this reaction also suggests avenues for further study, although the weight of present evidence militates against the implication of the C system in IgE-mediated histamine release.

Immune Complex Diseases

This term is currently used to describe an array of tissue injuries initiated by antigen-antibody aggregates formed in the fluid phase of reaction mixtures. As such, this term serves to differentiate fluid-phase events from the tissue damage which ensues after binding of the antigen to an immunoglobulin on a cell membrane. Since C activation by antigen and antibody always requires immune complexes and since fluid-phase and cellular events are often intimately related with respect to the nature of the tissue response, it seems that the term "immune complex disease" may be too inclusive and insufficiently informative of the immunopathological events caused by the interactions of antigen, antibody, and C. The discussion of the Arthus reaction which follows highlights the interplay of humoral and cellular reaction mechanisms.

ARTHUS REACTIONS

The phenomenon first described by Maurice Arthus at the turn of the century represents an excellent prototype of tissue injury caused by *in vivo* antigen-antibody aggregates. Many facets of the multiple-reaction mechanisms involved in the production of this form of immune vasculitis have been elucidated. A typical protocol for a passively induced Arthus reaction involves the intradermal inoculation of antibody which is immediately followed by an injection of antigen. Within three to four hours, the site of antibody deposition becomes indurated and hemorrhagic. The lesion is intensified during the next few hours and areas of necrosis develop by the next day. Microscopic examination reveals an early perivascular accumulation of neutrophils around the capillaries and venules. Fluorescent studies with the appropriate antisera reveal the presence of antigen, antibody, and C3 in the vessel walls. A similar histopathological response affecting the arteries occurs within the second week after a single injection of relatively large amounts of antigen intravenously. Various immune systems may be used to induce Arthus reactions provided the reactants are multivalent and capable of activating the C system via the classical or alternate pathways. The complex series of reactions leading to the vascular injury can be summarized as follows. The locally deposited immunoglobulins diffuse through the tissues and are aggregated by the antigen in the bloodstream. Antibody fixation to the tissues is not a prerequisite, but may occur. The immune complexes initiate the cascade of C-component interactions which lead to the generation of anaphylatoxins, and these chemotactic peptides induce a marked perivascular infiltration of polymorphonuclear leukocytes. In addition, the anaphylatoxins induce vascular permeability changes and enhance further deposition of the immune complexes. Phagocytosis of these aggregates by the neutrophils ensues, resulting in the release of lysosomal contents which include proteolytic enzymes. These destroy the integrity of the blood vessel walls through their attack on the vascular basement membrane, leading to the edema and hemorrhage of the Arthus reaction. Other products including low molecular weight (1000–4000 daltons) cationic peptides also contribute to these events.

Considerable emphasis has been placed on the roles of neutrophils and C in the pathogenesis of Arthus reactions. Thus deposits of antigen, antibody, and C3 have been identified in the vascular lesions. *In vivo* depletion of polymorphonuclear leukocytes or diminution of serum C activity with cobra venom suppresses the hemorrhage and necrosis without interfering with antigen-antibody deposition in the vascular endothelium. It is nevertheless difficult to understand why it has been concluded that platelets do not participate in the development of Arthus-type lesions in the rabbit. Seemingly all the conditions for thrombocytolysis, discussed in Chapter 7, are present. Moreover, earlier workers have described the presence of leukocyte-platelet-thrombi in the affected blood vessels, an observation fully consistent with the release of clotting factors from rabbit platelets under the impact of antigen-antibody complexes in a C-rich medium. While partial depletion of platelets does not influence the intensity of passively induced Arthus reactions, the immune vasculitis associated with active immunization of rabbits appears to require platelets.

The succession of these events has thus far been discussed in terms of the initiating immune complexes formed within the vascular system. The elicitation of the *active* Arthus reaction which depends on successive antigen injections and is a more physiological event probably leads to the presence of basophil-bound, antigen-specific IgE immunoglobulins. The role of these cell-bound reagins in the enhancement of tissue injury is discussed below in the section on Serum Sickness.

In summary, it is evident that the edema, hemorrhagic necrosis, and disruption of the vascular endothelium are manifestations of the biologic activities of C which emphasize the role of anaphylatoxins in mediating enhanced permeability, deposition of immune aggregates, leukotaxis, and release of lysosomal enzymes subsequent to phagocytosis.

SHWARTZMAN PHENOMENON

As is well known, this term is applied to the localized, dermal hemmorhagic necrosis which follows two injections of various lipopolysaccharides, one given locally and the second, intravenously twenty-four hours later. The many similarities of this response to the Arthus reaction were noted by Stetson, who inferred that the local reaction was mediated immunologically. This view did not receive general acceptance, the major reason being that this form of tissue damage could be induced nonspecifically, it seemed, through the use of two different and presumably unrelated lipopolysaccharides. The re-emergence of the alternate or properdin pathway of C activation and studies of its relationship to the Shwartzman reaction brought considerable clarity to this complex problem. Our understanding of the underlying mechanism was also extended by the findings of Heidelberger and of Springer pertaining to the extensive cross reactions among polysaccharide antigenic determinants. As a result, it is now generally accepted that normal animal sera usually contain specific immunoglobulins for many of the different lipopolysaccharides extracted from bacteria or fungi. Finally, the studies of Gewurz, discussed in Chapter 3, established that these endotoxins interact with the C system in two ways. The low antibody levels in normal sera bind the appropriate antigenic determinants and consume small but detectable quantities of C1, C4, and C2. The more significant finding relates to the disproportionate consumption of C3 and the late-acting components in a reaction mechanism dependent upon the alternate pathway. Both modes of C activation are probably set into motion when the lipopolysaccharides are injected into the skin. Anaphylatoxins are formed as a consequence of C utilization, leading to an influx of leukocytes, destruction of platelets, release of lysosomal hydrolases, and coagulation factors in a cascade of reactions closely simulating the events which ensue in the Arthus reaction. The second, intravenous injection of the same or a different lipopolysaccharide greatly amplifies these events and intensifies their tissue-damaging consequences at the local skin site.

The inference that antibodies in normal serum participate in the consumption of C1, C4, and C2 by endotoxin has been given material support in the experiments of Phillips and her collaborators, who identified a gamma-2 immunoglobulin as the mediating agent. In fact, Kane and others postulated that activation of the classical pathway was essential for the thrombocytopenia which results from the *in vivo* injection of endotoxin into guinea pigs. Further, the requirement for C6, demonstrated *in vitro* by Henson and *in vivo* by Fong and Good and by Johnson and Ward, suggests that in the rabbit, thrombocytolysis and endotoxin shock require utilization of the late-acting components, a consequence of both modes of C utilization. The release of coagulation factors from the disrupted platelets accounts for the leukocyte-platelet thrombi which are characteristic of the Shwartzman-type lesions. The varied results with sera from different mammals was stressed by Gewurz and his collaborators. They reported that C5a anaphylatoxin formation was most readily observed when bacterial lipopolysaccharides were incubated with pig or rat sera and, to a lesser extent, with mouse serum. The sera of humans, dogs, and cows did not support the generation of this peptide, suggesting that anaphylatoxin inhibitors may account for the apparently discrepant reports in the literature. In these experiments, detectable losses of C1, C4, and C2 were not found, again indicative of alternate pathway participation. Additional evidence for this interpretation was provided by the report of Marcus, Shin, and Mayer, who failed to detect a role for C2 in the degradation of C3 following incubation of an endotoxic lipopolysaccharide with guinea pig serum.

Poskitt, Fortwengler, and Lunskis have documented the interesting observation that red blood cell stroma activate the properdin pathway in autologous serum. Their conclusion is based on the formation of the C3 Activator ($\overline{B}$) from C3PA in these reactions. Intact erythrocytes, hemoglobin, and platelets are inactive. The authors suggest that intravascular damage to red blood cells by immune or other means may lead to activation of the alternate pathway and of the coagulation sequence through the release of platelet factor 3. These findings may therefore account for the syndrome of disseminated intravascular coagulation which occurs as a complication of acute hemolytic episodes. These events strongly resemble the generalized Shwartzman reaction which follows two intravenous inoculations of bacterial lipopolysaccharides in which the critical role of platelets has long been maintained by McKay. Activation of the alternate pathway in human serum by heterologous erythrocyte stroma has been demonstrated by Platts-Mills and Ishizaka.

SERUM SICKNESS

This type of immune complex disease which culminates in more generalized tissue damage often involving the vascular system and kidneys may be initiated by a single intravenous injection of a foreign protein in sufficient quantity. The experimental model in the rabbit has been studied extensively, and many aspects of the tissue-damaging processes have been elucidated over the past few decades. Following equilibration of the antigen in the intra- and extravascular spaces, the antigen is catabolized and disappears from the blood stream at a rate which varies with the nature of the heterologous protein. Within about one week, when the immune response has been elaborated to a sufficiently high degree, clearance of the antigen is accelerated, there is a fall in serum C levels, and manifestations of urticaria, fever, joint pains, arteritis, and glomerulonephritis become apparent. Histological studies show a marked accumulation of polymorphonuclear cells surrounding the arteries, with eventual destruction of the vascular endothelium and necrosis of the arterial wall. In large measure, the progression of these events recapitulates the reactions described above for the localized, passive Arthus phenomenon, with the additional finding of granular deposits in the glomeruli which account for the proteinuria and progressive renal damage. The use of isotopically labeled reagents show that these granular deposits contain the injected antigen, host antibody, and C3. The destructive effect of the immune complexes in the arterial walls is abrogated when the C levels of the animal are depleted by the prior injection of the cobra venom factor. A similar course of events may be initiated by the repetitive injection of small amounts of antigen over a period of a few weeks. The pathogenesis of this type of tissue injury has been well detailed by Cochrane and Koffler. Glomerulonephritis of the Masugi type may also be induced by the injection of a heterologous antiserum to renal tubular antigens.

An important question has been raised as to how the antigen-antibody complexes are deposited in the tissues as a prelude to the inflammatory and necrotic manifestations. With respect to the renal tissues, mechanical blockage by the basement membranes undoubtedly provides one means. Recent studies, however, provide strong support for the notion that the liberation of vasoactive compounds, possibly as a result of C3a and C5a formation, may be largely responsible for immune complex deposition. Direct evidence for this process was supplied by Benacerraf and his colleagues. These investigators injected colloidal carbon particles intravenously in mice which then received an injection of histamine, serotonin, epinephrine, or immune aggregates. Each of these agents caused the deposition of carbon in the intimal layers of large arteries, the walls of venules, and other sites. Cochrane extended these findings by showing that immune complex deposition was decreased by the presence of antihistamine or antiserotonin compounds. The biogenic amines could, of course, be released from platelets in the circulation and by the action of the C3a and C5a anaphylatoxins produced in the vascular system. There is, however, another means of platelet histamine release which is independent of the C system, and which is attributable to the synthesis of IgE following active immunization. As already mentioned, the IgE antibodies, bound to circulating basophils and tissue mast cells, react with their antigens and liberate histamine. In addition, these cells secrete a low molecular weight substance which liberates histamine and other vasoactive compounds from rabbit platelets. These agents undoubtedly enhance the tissue deposition of immune complexes and thereby contribute to the pathogenesis of tissue damage by antigen and antibody. Complexes which induce immune vasculitis are thought to have a molecular weight on the order of 7×10^6 daltons. Complexes in extreme antigen excess which may fail to activate C are also quite inactive in producing immune complex disease.

The pathogenesis of immune complex disease during active immunization also involves antibody fixation to monocyte and neutrophil membranes as well as to the vascular endothelium. The formation of immune aggregates on these surfaces as well as in the circulation leads to activation of the C system and the associated series of tissue-damaging events.

C AS A MEDIATOR OF TISSUE INJURY IN VIRAL INFECTIONS

The experimental models discussed above have their natural counterparts in glomerulonephritis caused by viral agents. This type of renal injury has been associated with a number of viral infections in which the disease process resembles the animal model of chronic serum sickness induced by repetitive injections of small amounts of foreign antigen over a period of weeks. These agents currently include the viruses of Moloney sarcoma, lymphocytic choriomeningitis, lactic dehydrogenase, Gross virus in New Zealand black mice, equine anemia, Aleutian disease of mink, and hog cholera. In each instance, the disease is characterized by the presence of granular deposits of host antibody and C along the glomerular capillary wall and mesangia, findings which are highly suggestive of immune complex disease.

Studies by Oldstone and Dixon of mice which are carriers of the lymphocytic choriomeningitis virus have provided firm evidence for a viral-induced immune complex disease and the possible genetic factors which influence the severity of the clinical manifestations. The results summarized in Table 9-1 illustrate the strain specificity which governs the incidence of

Table 9—1

Infectivity titers and immunofluorescent staining in
2- to 3-month-old lymphocytic choriomeningitis carrier mice *

	LD_{50} endpoint †	Intensity of staining for		
		LCM antigen	IgG	C3
SWR/J	5.4	+	++	++
B10D2 new	3.8	+	++	++
B10D2 old	3.6	+	++	++
NZB	3.4	+	++	++
AKR	2.0	+	±	±
C3H	1.6	+	±	±

* From M. B. A. Oldstone and F. J. Dixon, J. Exp. Med., **129**:487, 1969.
† Reciprocal of log dilution giving a 50% lethal endpoint with an inoculum isolated from mouse organs.

the carrier state and the identification of host antibody and C3 in the infected tissues.

As indicated in Table 9-1 the intensity of immunoreactant deposition could be correlated with the severity of the carrier state. Moreover, the circulating virus particles were found to be complexed with IgG and C3 since addition of the respective antibodies to the sera of carrier mice precipitated the virus. The glomerular basement membranes contained large amounts of IgG and C3, and significantly, eluates from the glomeruli of infected mice contained C-fixing antibodies for the LCM virion. It is not clear why the carrier state and immune complex disease do not occur readily in adult mice and why some strains are more vulnerable than others. Nor is it yet understood why infection and the carrier states induced by some viruses such as the lactic dehydrogenase agent are far less able to result in this form of C-mediated renal injury. In lymphocytic choriomeningitis, it has been postulated that the disease is most intense in those strains of mice which carry the heaviest virus burden and mount the greatest immune response. This variation in disease severity has been linked to the H-2 histocompatibility locus. It may not be amiss to suggest that the intensity of the immune response is but the forerunner of the degree of C activation.

Joseph and Oldstone have recently implicated the alternate C pathway in the lysis of Hela cells infected with measles virus. In the presence of specific antibody and C, Hela target cells which are infected with the measles virus are destroyed by antiviral antibody. These *in vitro* studies bear on the role of the alternate pathway since heating of the C source at 50° C for 20 minutes nullifies the cytotoxic activity which can be restored with purified C3PA.

Gocke and associates have offered substantial evidence to implicate the immunopathologic role of immune complexes in polyarteritis nodosa and hepatitis associated with chronic Australia antigenemia. The complexes found in the circulation contained the Australia antigen and immunoglobulins. C was also identified in deposits of these aggregates in the blood vessel walls.

The hemorrhagic shock syndrome frequently associated with group B arbovirus infection (Dengue hemorrhagic fever) provides another sample of C-mediated immunopathology. Studies by Bokisch and his colleagues showed that serum levels of all the classical C components, except for C9, as well as C3PA were depressed during shock. The fall in serum C levels was also associated with intravascular coagulation as deduced from the appearance of fibrinogen split products and thrombocytopenia. The rapid disappearance of C3 and its hypercatabolism in severely ill patients can be attributed to *in vivo* C utilization by virus-antibody complexes resulting in C3a and C5a anaphylatoxin formation. The vasoactive properties of the latter, i.e., histamine release and vasodilatation, probably contribute to the shock syndrome.

LEUKEMIA

A striking demonstration for the protective role of C5 in mouse leukemia was recently provided by the studies of Kassel, Old, and their colleagues. They found a marked reduction in the incidence of affected lymph nodes in AKR mice infused with normal heterologous sera. The protective factor was heat-labile and could be inactivated by heating to 56° C or treatment with cobra venom factor.

As shown in Fig. 9-1, the efficiency of the infusate depended on the presence of C5 in the donor's serum. Since the injection of purified C5, but

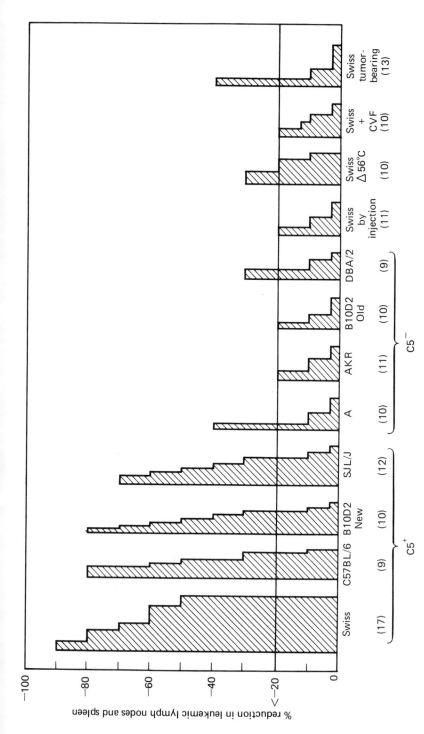

Fig. 9-1. AKR leukemic mice infused with normal serum from C5⁺ and C5⁻ mouse strains. Mice evaluated at 24 h postinfusion. Reduction >20% considered significant. Number in parenthesis indicates number of leukemic mice tested. Results: C5⁺ mouse serum causes reduction in leukemic lymph nodes and spleens. C5⁻ mouse serum is inactive. The antileukemic factor in Swiss mouse serum is (a) not demonstrable by injection (in contrast to infusion), (b) heat labile, (c) inactivated by CVF in vitro, and (d) reduced in tumor-bearing mice. (From R. L. Kassel, L. J. Old, E. A. Carswell, N. C. Fiore, and W. D. Hardy, Jr., *J. Exp. Med.*, **138:** 929, 1973.)

not of other C components, duplicated this effect, it would seem that the presence of viral antigens in the sera of leukemic AKR mice are also present in the transformed cells which then become susceptible to the cytotoxic action of C and antibody. The presence of these immunoreactants in the serum could therefore act as "enhancing factors" by diverting the C functions from the target cells. These findings are in accord with those of Ross and Polly, who identified receptors for inactivated C3, i.e., C3b on leukemic lymphoid cells in humans.

SYSTEMIC LUPUS ERYTHEMATOSUS (SLE)

Renal injury associated with this disease closely resembles chronic serum sickness caused by immune complexes. Serum C levels are markedly depressed during the active stages of SLE. Although many tissues may be affected, the extent of the lesions in the renal glomeruli and blood vessels greatly influences the course and outcome of the disease. In studies of the nature of the immune reactants associated with this disease, considerable emphasis has been placed on the finding that antibodies to host DNA may be found in the sera of SLE patients. In addition, the sera of these patients contain antibodies to a variety of cytoplasmic and nuclear constituents. From an etiologic viewpoint, it is of obvious importance to characterize the immunoreactants which initiate the process of cell destruction in SLE. Recent evidence suggests that a viral etiology may be involved. Very likely these and other antigens, aggregated by their specific antibodies, bind to cell membranes and activate the C system in a manner leading to cell injury and death. The cytoplasmic and nuclear constituents released into the circulation now stimulate further antibody production and tissue damage, in which glomerular insult is a prominent feature. Evidence strongly implicating immune complex deposition in the pathogenesis of this disease stems from the presence of DNA and other antigens, gamma globulins, and C components at the sites of glomerular damage. Significantly, immune globulins have been eluted from affected glomeruli. These antibodies were shown to react with native DNA, single-stranded DNA, and ribonucleoprotein.

In our studies with Townes and Stewart, a quantitative C-fixation procedure was used to estimate the quantity of immunoglobulins in the sera of SLE patients, capable of interaction with nucleoproteins, as described in Chapter 4. Serial assays over a period of months revealed a significant relationship between disease severity and the antinucleoprotein C-fixing capacity of the patient's serum. Moreover, C titrations with the same serum specimens indicated that the presence of antibody was associated with depressed C activity (see Figs. 9-2 and 9-3). These and other

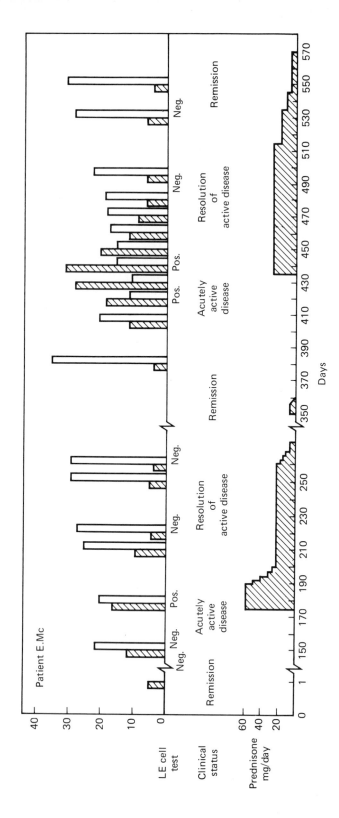

Fig. 9-2. Variations in levels of serum C and nucleoprotein-reactive gamma globulin with clinical course and treatment. (From A. S. Townes, C. R. Stewart, Jr., and A. G. Osler, *Bull. Johns Hopkins Hospital*, **112**:212, 1963.)

Nucleoprotein reactive gamma globulin μg N/ml

Serum complement, CH_{50}/ml

Patient E.Mc

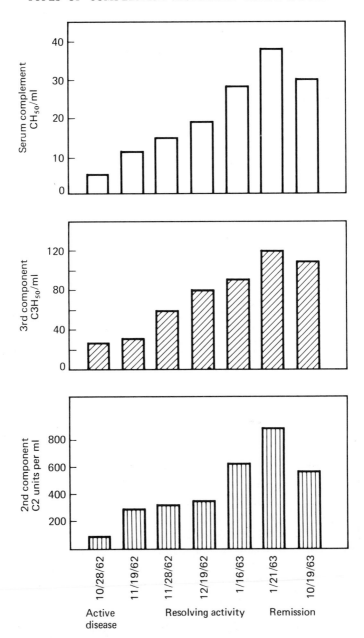

Fig. 9-3. Estimations of C, C2, and C3 during the course of SLE in Patient E. H. (From A. S. Townes and C. R. Stewart, Jr., *Bull. Johns Hopkins Hospital,* **117:**353, 1965.)

observations suggest that the pronounced *in vivo* utilization of C1, C4, C2, and C3 account for the low serum C levels. Moreover, the deposition of C3 in the renal tissues of SLE patients and the finding that serum levels of the late C components are inversely related to disease severity, as shown in Fig. 9-4, point to the important role of C in the pathogenesis of tissue damage in SLE. Convincing evidence is available to substantiate the pres-

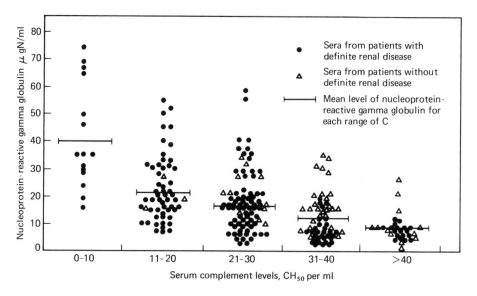

Fig. 9-4. Serum complement and nucleoprotein-reactive gamma globulin values in 248 sera from 35 patients with systemic lupus erythematosus. (From A. S. Townes, C. R. Stewart, Jr., and A. G. Osler, *Bull. Johns Hopkins Hospital,* **112:205,** 1963.)

ence of immune complexes in the sera of SLE patients. These sera are often anticomplementary in the sense that they consume the hemolytic activity of fresh serum upon admixture and incubation. Tissue deposits of immunoglobulins and antigens, as well as of C3, have been identified. The circulating complexes can be precipitated upon the addition of C1q. In addition, Vyas has shown that the sera of 22 of 25 SLE patients will inhibit the uptake of radioiodinated HSA-anti-HSA complexes by guinea pig peritoneal exudate cells. In the study by Vyas, sera of normal individuals failed to inhibit the competitive uptake of the HSA immune aggregates. Further, treatment of the SLE sera with DNase abrogated the inhibition. Although the circumstantial evidence is striking, the nature of the immune complexes with respect to the class of immunoglobulins, the ratios of antibody to antigen, the nature of the determinants, their specific C-fixing potencies, the presence of C-cleavage products at the lesion site, and the glomerular or mesangial localization of the various immunoreactants are all factors which may influence the activation of C and the resulting clinical picture.

Since active immunization undoubtedly sets the stage for the widespread clinical manifestations of SLE, one may reasonably assume that IgE synthesis also occurs and intensifies the binding of other immune aggregates to the affected tissues as discussed above in relation to immune complex disease. In addition, the participation of cellular immune mechanisms has been invoked in the mediation of renal tissue injury without implicating C activation. A recent report indicates that the activity levels of all the C components except C1 are diminished in male guinea pigs following injection of 100 mg/kg of cortisone acetate for two weeks. It is doubtful that these changes alone are of sufficient magnitude to account for the amelioration of symptoms in SLE by this steroid.

The participation of the properdin pathway in the pathogenesis of SLE may be inferred from the reports of Perrin and others, who found decreased serum levels of properdin and Factor B, and of Day and others, who identified properdin in the renal basement membrane of patients with this multisystem, immunologic disease. The latter group also found an association between C2 deficiency and SLE. They postulated that this C deficiency accounted for the repetitive infections which plague these patients and which may account for the subsequent development of SLE.

HYPOCOMPLEMENTIC GLOMERULONEPHRITIS

This type of renal damage is of interest since its study by West, Spitzer, Vallota, and their colleagues revealed several features of immunologic interest. Although antigen-antibody aggregates have not been implicated, immunofluorescent staining identified deposits of immunoglobulins and C3 in the glomeruli with basement membrane alterations. Serum C levels are depressed, the deficit being due to low C3 without significant diminution of C1, C4, or C2. The sera of patients with this disease contain C3 fragments, notably the a-2D antigen and a factor capable of cleaving C3 in the presence of magnesium, called C3NeF. Like the situation in SLE, this type of nephritis is frequently associated with glomerular deposition of properdin at sites which also contain C3. These findings and the failure as yet to implicate immune complexes suggest that activation of the alternate pathway constitutes the major immunopathological process. However, the presence of immunoglobulin deposits as well as of C1q and C4 in the glomeruli militates against exclusion of the classical route of C activation as a contributory mechanism. In fact, the C3NeF, nephritic factor, has recently been isolated from the sera of patients with this disease and has been shown to require Factors B and D for the fragmentation of C3. It has been identified as a 7S globulin with a molecular weight of 150,000 daltons which behaves electrophoretically as a gamma globulin. It does not activate the classical pathway. In this sense it differs from the cobra venom factor. It partakes in the cleavage of C3 with anaphylatoxin production in the presence of Factor B, C3PAse (Factor D), and magnesium. Antiserum to C3NeF removes a normal serum constituent which may function as an inactive precursor of C3NeF. C3NeF is not considered to be an immunoglobulin but may cleave C3 in a manner analogous to the action of properdin.

RHEUMATOID ARTHRITIS

The inclusion of this disease under the heading of immune complex disease can be readily justified in terms of its pathogenetic mechanism. Elucidation of the immunopathologic sequence has emerged from studies of the lesion site, the synovial membrane, and the joint fluids. One of the early findings was that hemolytic complement levels were reduced in rheumatoid synovial fluids, as compared with inflammatory lesions due to other causes. This depression is due to activation of the classical and alternate pathways leading to a reduction in the levels of C4, C2, and C3. The joint fluids of rheumatoid arthritis patients contain the trimolecular complex C567 as well as the C3 convertase, $\overline{C42}$, and C3 fragments. Components of the alternate pathway are also present in synovial fluids. Studies in our laboratory with about forty specimens provided by Dr. Alex Townes showed marked fluctuations in hemolytic activity levels of Factor B, but no definite pattern emerged which could be correlated with the clinical features of the disease. However, as shown in Table 9-2, C3PA levels correlated well with

Table 9–2

Average values for complement and the C3 activator system in synovial fluid from various forms of arthritis *

Form of arthritis	No. of patients	Protein (g %)	CH_{50}	C3PA (μg/ml)	C3A
Rheumatoid arthritis	9	4.75	15	86	3/9
Infectious arthritis	6	5.75	120	213	3/6
Inflammatory (non-RA) arthritis	9	5.09	87	196	0/9
Osteoarthritis	4	3.97	45	88	0/4

* From N. J. Zvaifler, Arth. and Rheumatism, 17:301, 1974.

total hemolytic activity of these fluids. The leukocytes in synovial fluids like those in SLE have cytoplasmic inclusions of immunoglobulin and C components. The chemotactic factors generated by C activation, such as C5a and C567, are probably responsible for the continued influx of large numbers of polymorphonuclear cells. Zvaifler has estimated that as many as 300 million neutrophils may pass through the articular cavity in a single day. The extrusion of lysosomal hydrolases following phagocytosis of the immune complexes in the joint may therefore be primarily responsible for the inflammation and tissue destruction which characterize this disease. An additional factor to be considered in evaluating the immunological events which take place within the synovia has been brought to light by Ruddy and Colten. They showed that rheumatoid synovial tissues synthesize C2, C3, C4, and C5 to a far greater extent than do these tissues derived from patients with degenerative or traumatic arthritis. As in SLE, the initial immune events which set this sequence into motion are not known. There is, however, conclusive evidence that immune complexes containing the 7S and 19S rheumatoid factors are present in synovial fluids of patients with this disease. They have been demonstrated by such assays as C fixation, histamine release, precipitation on the addition of IgM rheumatoid factor, C1q cryoprecipitation, ultracentrifugation, and the induction of leukotaxis. Some investigators consider that the presence of these immune complexes results from an autoimmune response in the synovial tissues to antigenic determinants present on host tissues and gamma globulins which are released following the localized tissue destruction. Components which may provide these antigenic determinants include fibrin, leukocytic nucleoprotein, denatured DNA, etc. The demonstration that as much as 95 mg of IgG can be produced within the synovium in a single day is fully consistent with this concept. For a time, the role of C in these events was questioned in view of the demonstration that some IgM rheumatoid factors are unable to activate the C system. This difficulty was technical in nature since the use of aggregated gamma globulins as antigens renders difficult the interpretation of C-fixation assays because they are highly anticomplementary. However, reduction and alkylation of these aggregates uncovered their pronounced C-fixing potencies with rheumatoid factors. Elevated titers of the rheumatoid factors have been well correlated with their C-fixing capacities as well as with disease severity.

Enhanced C Activity Levels

The complement literature contains a number of reports attesting to an increased hemolytic C activity in the sera of patients with a variety of disorders. More than twenty years ago, Fishel documented a rise in C1 associated with acute inflammatory reactions such as myocardial infarctions. Nishioka has reviewed more recent studies in which elevated hemolytic activity levels of serum C were observed in the sera of tumor-bearing animals and humans with neoplastic disease. Similar findings apply to the alternate pathway. Studies of C3 proactivator levels in our laboratory, as assayed by the cobra-venom-mediated lysis of unsensitized red blood cells, showed elevated levels of this properdin system reactant in the sera of human cancer patients. The titers of sera furnished by healthy adults and by patients hospitalized with a variety of non-neoplastic diseases were generally lower than those of patients with malignant tumors. The titer distribution profiles also set the cancer patients apart from the other two groups in that values above 30 hemolytic units per ml occurred about eight times more frequently in the cancer group. These observations were extended with similar results to the sera of mice bearing tumors induced by 3-methylcholanthrene. Here too, the serum titers of cancerous mice were significantly higher $(P < 0.001)$ than those in concurrently maintained healthy controls. Further, the serum titers of mice injected with the carcinogen but which failed to develop tumors fell within the normal range. Neither sex nor body weight at time of bleeding proved to be significant variables. The titer increase was, however, correlated with splenomegaly and tumor weight.

Pregnancy in the human is likewise associated with increased C3PA activity levels. The mean titer for the sera of 54 pregnant women was 46.7 ± 8.5 as compared with that of the control group $(n = 43)$ which was 30.5 ± 7.9, $P < 0.001$. A bar graph illustrating these results is given in Fig. 9-5. Of interest is the observation that the mean value observed in pregnancy was indistinguishable from that of 39 cancer patients' sera, i.e., 43.7 ± 8.4. The elevation of C3PA titers occurred primarily in the third trimester of gestation and persisted for at least one week during the postnatal period.

Higher serum levels of hemolytic complement and of C4, C3, and C3 Activator were recently found in patients with juvenile rheumatoid arthritis, as compared to age- and sex-matched healthy controls. The significance of these increases in C activity is suggested by the report showing similar changes in the sera of rats following immunization with antigen emulsified in Freund's complete adjuvant or with the adjuvant itself. The rise in C activity was localized to an increase in the first six components of the classical pathway during the first three weeks of immunization. C and component titers then gradually returned to normal levels. In this sense the several C components resemble the C-reactive protein as acute phase reactants.

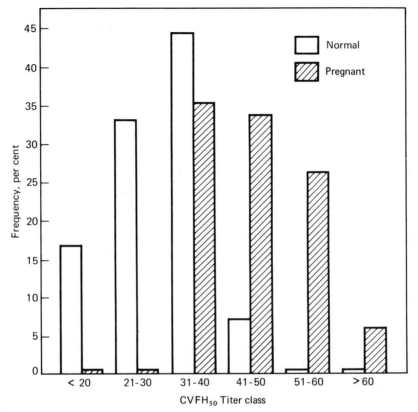

Fig. 9-5.

Nonimmune Mechanisms of C Activation

A number of nonimmune reaction systems capable of C activation have been described. Several such as those involving polynucleotides, complexes of lysozyme with single-stranded DNA, and heparin with protamine are of theoretical interest in that they may contribute to an understanding of the molecular requirements of C activation mechanisms. These observations may also be pertinent to studies of C in immunopathology as potential recognition factors in host-defense mechanisms. One of these, discussed in Chapter 4, deals with C activation through the interaction of staphylococcal Protein A with the Fc fragment of IgG. The consequences of this mode of C utilization include platelet lysis, leukotaxis, and the production of Arthus-type lesions in the rabbit. Following the publication of these reports, it has been observed that streptococcal and pneumococcal constituents can also activate C in their reactions with the Fc fragment. In the case of the pneumococci, the available evidence favored the participation of the polysaccharide component in the nonimmune C fixation with the Fc portion of the immunoglobulins. Volanakis and Kaplan recently described an interesting example of this type. They observed that crystalline C-reactive protein or sera containing this acute phase reactant fixed C via the classical pathway when incubated with the pneumococcal C polysaccharide. Marked consumption of C1, C4, and C2, as well as of C3–C9, characterized this process. The reaction was completely inhibited by phosphoryl choline, the major antigenic determinant of the C-reactive protein but not by N-acetyl galactosamine. Sera lacking the C-reactive protein were inactive. C fixation was not observed when guinea pig serum was added to the C-reactive protein, the failure being traced to the inactivity of guinea pig C1q in this reaction. The consequences of C consumption by complexes of C-reactive protein and human C components like that of the staphylococcal A protein indicates the potential role of this form of nonimmune activation in inflammation.

FURTHER READING

Cochrane, C. G., and Koffler, D., "Immune Complex Disease in Experimental Animals and Man," *Adv. Immunol.,* **16**:185, 1973.

Immune Complexes and Disease, Several Pertinent Articles in *J. Exp. Med.,* **134**: No. 3, Part 2, 1971.

Leber, P. D., and McCluskey, R. T., "Complement and the Immunohistology of Renal Disease," *Trans. Proc.,* **6**:67, 1974.

McLean, R. H., and Michael, A. F., "Properdin and C3 Proactivator: Alternate Pathway Components in Human Glomerulonephritis," *J. Clin. Invest.,* **52**:634, 1973.

Vallota, E. H., Götze, O., Spiegelberg, H. L., Forristal, J., West, C. D., and Müller-Eberhard, H. J., "A Serum Factor in Chronic Hypocomplementemic Nephritis Distinct From Immunoglobulins and Activating The Alternate Pathway of Complement," *J. Exp. Med.,* **139**:1249, 1974.

Volanakis, J. E., and Kaplan, M. H., "Interaction of C-Reactive Protein Complexes with the Complement System," *J. Immunol.,* **113**:9, 1974.

Wilson, C. B., and Dixon, F. J., "Immunopathology and Glomerulonephritis," *Ann. Rev. Medicine,* **25**:83, 1974.

Zvaifler, N. J., "The Immunopathology of Joint Inflammation in Rheumatoid Arthritis," *Adv. Immunol.,* **16**:265, 1973.

Index

A

ADP, and platelet agglutination, 145

agglutinins, cold and warm, 130

alexin, 1

allergic reactions (*see also* immunoglobulins, IgE):

due to reaginic and nonreaginic immunoglobulins, 4–5

allogeneic transplants, and humoral antibody, 138

allograft reactions, 137

allograft survival, role of the alternate pathway, 139

alternate complement pathways, 32–55 (*see also* properdin system)

activation of, 41–53

in anaphylatoxin production, 151

antibody synthesis, 123, 126

compared to classical C pathway, 47

dysfunction, 105

in hypocomplementic glomerulonephritis, 179

in invertebrate hemolymph, 92

lysis of nucleated cells, 135

lysis of viral infected cells, 173

in opsonization, 111

and phagocytosis, 113

platelet histamine release, 144

alternate complement pathways (*cont.*)

platelet lysis, 144

platelet serotonin release, 146

in Shwartzman reaction, 168

in SLE, 179

anaphylatoxins, 5, 128, 164 (*see also* C3a and C5a)

biologic properties, 152–9

formation and characterization, 149–52

generation in Arthus reaction, 167

inhibitor of, 150

and lysosomal enzyme release, 115

in Shwartzman reaction, 169

anaphylaxis, 3, 129

antibody:

lysis mediated by, 12

reactivity of, from different species, 12

synthesis, 123

antigen:

assay by C fixation, 73

detection on cell surfaces by C̄IFT, 76

antigen-antibody complexes, activation of the alternate pathway, 44

antilymphocyte serum, 139

antiplatelet antibody, 140

antrypol, 24, 26, 30
Arthus reaction, 167
autoantibodies, 129–34

B

bactericidal reactions, 107–10
  due to alternate pathway activation, 108
bacteriolysis, 107–8
  requirement for nine C components, 108
basophils, chemotactic factors for, 157
blood coagulation, 159
bradykinin, 151, 160

C

C-reactive protein, 163, 184
cell membrane, 26–8
  lesions produced by C action, 26, 110
  lipid mosaic model of, 26
cellular intermediates of immune hemolysis:
  EA, 15, 18
  EAC1, 17–19
  EAC14, 76
  EAC14b, 17–19
  EAC142, 18, 132
    decay, 58
  EAC1423, 132
  EAC4, 19, 76
  EAC42, 19
  EAC423, 20–2
  EAC4235, 23
  EAC423567, 22
classical complement system, 6–31
  comparison with alternate C pathway, 47

cobra venom factor:
  activation of the alternate pathway, 49–52
    compared to other methods of activation, 50
  activation of invertebrate hemolymph, 92
  anticomplementary action, 49
  characterization, 49
  complex formation with Factors B and D, 49–51
  destruction of C3, 37, 49
    effect on antibody synthesis, 123
cold agglutinin syndrome, 132
complement activation:
  comparison of classical and properdin system, 47
  nonimmune mechanisms, 13, 53, 183
complement components:
  biosynthesis of, 85–92
  measurement of, 14
  metabolism of, 94
  physiochemical properties, 7
complement fixation, 56–83
  aggregation of antibody, 70–1
  antigen assays by, 73–6
  comparative potencies of 7S and 19S immunoglobulins, 77
  for estimate of relative antibody content, 60, 68
  five CH50 unit method, 67
  methods, limitations, 68
  micro method, 65–7
  multivalency of antigen, 70
  nature of the antigen, 72
  properties of the immune complex, 69–72
  quantitative, 68
  techniques, 65
complement receptor lymphocytes, 120–2

complement receptors, on polymorphonuclear leukocytes and macrophages, 114
conglutinin, 3, 30, 38
conglutinogen-activating factor (*see* C3b inactivator*)
cyclic AMP, and release of histamine, 165
cytolysis, 134
  mechanism of, 26
  sensitivity to and cell cycle, 134
cytotoxic reactions, 4
cytotoxicity, C-mediated, 128–48
C1, 20
  activation by kallikrein, 97, 159
  activation by plasmin, 97, 159
  assembly and action, 14–17
  binding to aggregated immunoglobulins, 76
  biosynthesis, 85, 87
  fixation and transfer test, 19, 76
    applications, 76, 130
  on red cell membranes, *in vivo,* 132
  rise in acute inflammatory reactions, 182
  and virus neutralization, 117, 119
C1q, 7, 15–17
  binding to immunoglobulins, 11, 62
  deficiency of, 96
  metabolism, 94
C1r, 7, 15–16
  deficiency of, 96
C1s, 7, 15
C1 esterase, in hereditary angioedema, 97
C1 esterase inhibitor, phylogenetic studies, 92, 94
C1 inactivator, 8 [*see also* C1 Inh (C1 inhibitor)]
C1 INH (C1 inhibitor), 8, 16, 18
  and blood coagulation, 160
  concentration in serum, 97

C1 INH (*cont.*)
  deficiency of, 96
  leukotaxis enhancement, 157
  site of action, 29
C1 inhibitors, 16–17
  DFP, 16
C2, 7, 17
  in the assembly of C3 convertase, 18
  biosynthesis, 88
  deficiency in man, 100
  depletion in hereditary angioedema, 97
  synthesis by rheumatoid synovial tissues, 181
  and virus neutralization, 117, 119
C2-dependent permeability factor, 159
C3, 7, 18, 172
  binding to erythrocytes, 130
  binding to erythrocytes of patients with PNH, 49
  biosynthesis, 86, 88
  cell bound and hemolytic anemia, 132
  deficiency of:
    in guinea pigs, 101
    in man, 101
  depletion and antibody synthesis, 123
  estimation of, 79
  estimation of cell bound C3 by $C\overline{1}FT$, 79
  genetic polymorphism of, 101
  hydrazine sensitive factor, 37
  hypercatabolism of, 36
    type-1 essential hypercatabolism of, 105
  inactivation by zymosan, 32
  inhibitors (*see also* C3b inactivator):
    hydrazine, 37, 150
    phlorizin, 150, 164

C3 (*cont.*)
  lymphocyte receptors, 12
  metabolism, 95
  and opsonic activity, 113
  in opsonization, 111
  participation in thymus-dependent immune response, 123
  and phagocytosis, 111
  receptor on monocytes, 115
  requirement in immune adherence, 81
  structure, 20
  synthesis by rheumatoid synovial tissues, 181
  tissue deposits in SLE, 178
  and virus neutralization, 117, 119
C3a, 149, 163 (*see also* anaphylatoxins)
  formation of, 21
  formation in serum sickness, 171
  properties and structure of human, 151
C3b, 145
  feedback mechanism in properdin pathway, 38, 44
  formation of, 20, 21
  in immune adherence, 111
  participation in properdin pathway, 38, 39, 40, 44
  receptor on leukemic lymphoid cells in humans, 175
  receptor on lymphocytes, 121
  receptor on phagocytes, 114
  zymosan bound, 43
C3c, 21, 30, 38
C3d, 21, 38
  receptor on lymphocytes, 121
  receptor on phagocytes, 114
C3 convertase:
  decay, 19, 29
  formation of, 18–20
C3b inactivator, 8, 21

C3b inactivator (*cont.*)
  deficiency of, 105, 106
  proteolysis of C3b, 38
  site of action, 29
  structure and characterization, 29
C3 Nef (C3 nephritic factor), 179
  characterization, 180
  cleavage of C3, 180
  role in properdin system, 38
C3 proactivator (C3PA), 134, 170, 180 (*see also* Factor B)
  characterization, 37
  complex formation with cobra venom factor, 37, 49
  elevation in sera:
    in cancer patients, 182
    in human pregnancy, 182
C3PAse (*see* Factor D)
C4, 7, 17
  biosynthesis, 88
  deficiency in guinea pigs, 98
  deficiency in man, 98
  deficiency in rats, 100
  depletion in hereditary angioedema, 97
  quantitation of cell bound C4, 80
  structure, 17
  substrate for $C\overline{1}$, 17, 18
  synthesis by rheumatoid synovial tissues, 181
  and virus neutralization, 117, 119
C4a, 17, 158
C4 deficient guinea pigs, 129
C4 inactivator, 8
C5, 7, 139, 150
  biosynthesis, 89
  deficiency of
    in man, 104
    in mice, 103
  in lytic sequence, 22–5
  and phagocytosis, 113
  proteolytic cleavage, 23, 24

C5 (*cont.*)
  synthesis by rheumatoid synovial
    tissues, 181
C5a, 23, 149–59, 163 (*see also* ana-
    phylatoxins)
  formation in serum sickness, 171
  properties of human, 151
  structure, 151
C5 convertase:
  decay, 21, 29
  formation of, 20
C567
  binding site for C8, 23
  chemotactic factor for neutro-
    phils, 155, 181
  in joint fluid of rheumatoid ar-
    thritis patients, 180
  trimolecular complex, 22, 23, 155
C6, 7, 139
  biosynthesis, 92
  in blood coagulation, 160
  deficiency:
    in man, 105
    in rabbits, 104
  in lytic sequence, 22
C6 inactivator, 8
  site of action, 30
C7, 7, 139
  in lytic sequence, 22
C8, 7, 139
  binding to C567, 23
  in lytic sequence, 22
C9, 7
  binding and activity, 23
  biosynthesis, 92
  in lytic sequence, 22

D

defense mechanisms, C mediated,
    107–27

E

EGTA, suppression of classical C
    pathway, 42
endotoxic lipopolysaccharide, 168
  activation of the properdin path-
    way, 41, 47, 50
eosinophils, chemotactic factors for,
    157
epsilon-aminocaproic acid, 150
erythrocytes:
  K+ content and susceptibility to
    lysis, 13
  resistance to antibody mediated
    lysis, 12
erythrophagocytosis, 113, 130

F

Factor A, 37 (*see also* C3)
Factor B, 36–40, 43, 47, 158 (*see
    also* C3 proactivator)
  activation, 38
  C3 cleavage by, 37–9, 47
  characterization, 36, 40
  hemolytic assay, 51
  identity with GBG, C3PA, 36
  interaction with cobra venom fac-
    tor, 49–51
  polymorphism, 105
Factor B convertase (*see* Factor D)
Factor D, 36
  activation, 38
  characterization, 38
  inhibition, 38
  complex formation with CVF and
    C3PA, 50
Factor E, role in lysis of unsensitized
    erythrocytes, 51
F(ab')₂ fragment, 63

F(ab')₂ fragment (*cont.*)
  alternate pathway activation, 45,
    111
Fc piece:
  activation of classical C pathway,
    45, 62
  binding to C1q, 16, 62
Forssman antigen, 4, 10
Forssman shock, 128

G

GBG (*see* Factor B)
GBGase, 36 (*see also* Factor D)
GBGase inhibitor, 36
genetics of the C system, 95–106
glomerulonephritis, 170
  caused by viral agents, 171
graft rejection, 137–40

H

H2 locus, 91, 122
  and synthesis of C, 87
Hageman factor, and C1 activation,
    97, 159
hemolymph, activation by cobra
    venom factor, 92
hemolysis, immune:
  dose-response curve, 57–8
  parameters influencing the reac-
    tion, 9
  in vivo:
    mediated by C and "autoanti-
      bodies," 129–34
    mediated by C in the absence
      of antibody, 134
hemolytic anemia, 129, 132

hemolytic C titers, hormonal influ-
    ence, in mice, 89–91
hemorrhagic shock syndrome, 173
hereditary angioedema, 96
histamine:
  release of, 3–5, 171
    by anaphylatoxins, 152
  release by IgE, 78, 165, 171
    in PCA, 163
  release by platelets, 140–7
hydrazine, inhibition of C3, C4, 37
hypocomplementic glomerulonephri-
    tis, 179

I

immune adherence, 80, 111
immune aggregates, C fixation by
    preformed, 44, 50
immune complex diseases, 166–81
immunoconglutinin, 30
immunoglobulins:
  affinity, 60
  binding of C1q, 58, 61
  C-fixing sites on, 61
  class and subclasses in human
    serum, 10
  differences in C activation, 10
  IgA, 11
    activation of the alternate path-
      way, 60
    and phagocytosis, 114
  IgE, 11, 61, 146, 164, 171
    allergic reactions mediated by,
      4, 165
    sites on basophils, 78
  IgG, 4, 11, 59, 164, 172
    C-fixation, compared to IgM,
      58
    cytotoxic reactions, 4
    estimation of cell bound, 130

immunoglobulins, IgG (*cont.*)
  hemolytic capacity, 11
  and phagocytosis, 114
  receptor on monocytes, 115
  IgG1, guinea pig, 5, 10
    activation of the alternate pathway, 44
    C activation by F(ab')$_2$ fragment, 45
    failure to mediate passive immune hemolysis, 63
    in PCA reaction, 165
  IgG2, guinea pig, 10
    C activation by F(ab')$_2$ and Fc, 45
    C fixation compared to IgG1, 44
    in phagocytosis, 111
  IgM:
    C fixation, compared to IgG, 58
    cytotoxic reactions, 4
    estimation of cell bound, 130
    hemolytic capacity, 10
    and phagocytosis, 114
inflammation, 149–61
inhibitors of C components (*see* "inactivators" under individual C components)
inulin, activation of the alternate pathway, 44, 47, 50

K

K antigen, and susceptibility to C mediated destruction, 108
KAF (*see* C3b inactivator)
kallikrein, 29, 97, 159
kinins, 158
  in C1 activation, 97

L

leukemia, protective role of C5, 173
leukotaxis, 153
liposomes, 28
lymphocytic choriomeningitis, 172
lysosomal enzymes, release of, by C5a, 157
lysozyme, 110
  role in spheroplast formation, 108

M

macrophages, "activated," 115
metal requirements, classical and alternate pathway, 47
mononuclear cells, chemotactic factors for, 157
Mu B1 antigen, 103

N

neutrophils, chemotactic factors for, 155

O

one-hit theory, 1, 8–10, 14, 26, 58
ontogenetic development of the C system, 85–92
opsonic activity, 113
opsonization, 111

P

paroxysmal nocturnal hemoglobinuria, 134
  lysis of erythrocytes, 32, 34, 48, 49

passive cutaneous anaphylaxis (PCA,), 163
   in the guinea pig, 164
   in the mouse, 165
   in the rat, 164
phagocytosis, 110–16
   of erythrocytes, 113, 130
   facilitation by C5, 113
   by macrophages, 114
   participation of the alternate pathway, 111
   by polymorphonuclear leukocytes, 114
phylogeny of the C system, 92–4
platelet:
   activating factor (PAF), 146
   agglutination, 145
   immunologic mechanisms of damage, 145, 169
   lysis 140–7, 160
      by C and antibody, 140
      by unrelated antigen-antibody complexes (allergic type), 142–7
properdin, 32
   characterization, 34
   radioimmunoassay of, 34
properdin system, 32–55 (see also alternate complement pathways)
   activation of, 41–9
   bactericidal action, 108
   components, 34–40
      properties of, 41
      mode of action, 39
   dysfunction, 105
protein A from staphylococcus aureus, 3, 183
   complement fixation by, 81
   biologic consequences of protein A-serum interaction, 83

R

reactive lysis, 22, 139
reaginic allergy, 3 (see also immunoglobulins, IgE)
receptors:
   for C on lymphocytes, 120–3
   for Fc fragment on lymphocytes, 121
rheumatoid arthritis, 180
rheumatoid factors, 3

S

salicylaldoxime, inhibitor of alternate pathway, 47
serotonin:
   release of, 152
   release from human platelets, 146
serum sickness, 170
Shwartzman phenomenon, 168–70
sickle-cell disease, deficiency in phagocytosis, 116
smooth muscle contraction, by C3a and C5a, 153
staphylococcus protein A (see protein A from staphylococcus aureus)
systemic lupus erythematosus (SLE), 175–9

T

thrombocytolysis (see platelet, lysis)
thrombocytopenia, 140, 146
tissue injury:
   antibody mediated, 4
   C associated, 162–84

tissue injury (*cont.*)
  in viral infections, 171–3

V

virus-antibody complexes, 171–3
virus neutralization, enhancement by
      C, 116–20
virus transformed cells, fixation of
      C by, 134

W

Wasserman test for syphilis, 2

X

xenografts, 138

Z

zymosan:
  activation of properdin pathway,
      41–3
  C3 cleaving enzyme on, 43
  C5 cleaving enzyme on, 43
  destruction of C3 by, 32
  and platelet serotonin release, 146